SpringerBriefs in Well-Being and Quality of Life Research

SpringerBriefs in Well-Being and Quality-of-Life Research are concise summaries of cutting-edge research and practical applications across the field of well-being and quality of life research. These compact refereed monographs are under the editorial supervision of an international Advisory Board*. Volumes are 50 to 125 pages (approximately 20,000–70,000 words), with a clear focus. The series covers a range of content from professional to academic such as: snapshots of hot and/or emerging topics, in-depth case studies, and timely reports of state-of-the art analytical techniques. The scope of the series spans the entire field of Well-Being Research and Quality-of-Life Studies, with a view to significantly advance research. The character of the series is international and interdisciplinary and will include research areas such as: health, cross-cultural studies, gender, children, education, work and organizational issues, relationships, job satisfaction, religion, spirituality, ageing from the perspectives of sociology, psychology, philosophy, public health and economics in relation to Well-being and Quality-of-Life research. Volumes in the series may analyze past, present and/or future trends, as well as their determinants and consequences. Both solicited and unsolicited manuscripts are considered for publication in this series. SpringerBriefs in Well-Being and Quality-of-Life Research will be of interest to a wide range of individuals with interest in quality of life studies, including sociologists, psychologists, economists, philosophers, health researchers, as well as practitioners across the social sciences. Briefs will be published as part of Springer's eBook collection, with millions of users worldwide. In addition, Briefs will be available for individual print and electronic purchase. Briefs are characterized by fast, global electronic dissemination, standard publishing contracts, easy-to-use manuscript preparation and formatting guidelines, and expedited production schedules. We aim for publication 8–12 weeks after acceptance.

Robert A. Stebbins

Project-Based Leisure

Toward Personal Well-Being and Community
Involvement

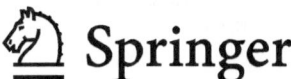 Springer

Robert A. Stebbins 🆔
Department of Sociology
University of Calgary
CALGARY, AB, Canada

ISSN 2211-7644   ISSN 2211-7652   (electronic)
SpringerBriefs in Well-Being and Quality of Life Research
ISBN 978-3-031-47051-6   ISBN 978-3-031-47052-3   (eBook)
https://doi.org/10.1007/978-3-031-47052-3

This Springer imprint is published by the registered company Springer Nature Switzerland AG
The registered company address is: Gewerbestrasse 11, 6330 Cham, Switzerland

Paper in this product is recyclable.

Preface

For many people, there are times in everyday life that are available for leisure, though not large enough or frequent enough to enable pursuing a serious hobby, amateur activity, or major volunteer role. Some people fill these temporal interstices—the small gaps between work, non-work obligations, and enduring casual and serious leisure interests—with *project-based leisure* (PBL). These activities, which may be spontaneous, help round out our leisure lifestyle. PBL is a short-term, reasonably complicated, one-off, or occasional, though infrequent, creative, or inventive undertaking carried out in free time, or time free of disagreeable obligation. Such leisure may require considerable planning, effort, and sometimes skill or knowledge (Stebbins 2005). Yet, it is not serious leisure nor initially intended to develop into such.

In other words, PBL contributes to our subjective well-being, though doing so more modestly than serious leisure and occupational devotion. Without it we either resort in these interstices to casual leisure or return to life's obligations (i.e., disagreeable work and non-work activities). In these options, subjective well-being is reduced accordingly. Note that project-based leisure cannot, by definition, refer to projects executed as part of a person's serious leisure. Examples include routinely mounting community star nights as an amateur astronomer or model train displays as a hobbyist collector.

Nonetheless, PBL can generate a sense of satisfaction, of having accomplished something, if nothing else of having an agreeable experience that is out of the ordinary. Completing a jigsaw puzzle or watching an educational video exemplify such leisure, so long as they are one-off activities or, at most, infrequently done. In this fashion PBL contributes to our well-being.

Project-based leisure is a relatively new idea in the serious leisure perspective, which however, has already generated some field research. According to the

Bibliography at www.seriousleisure.net, 23 studies have been conducted on PBL since 2005. The idea has resonated well with leisure studies scholars, even while additional clarification of the original statement is in order. That clarification is the goal of this monograph, which will be achieved in part with reference to these studies.

Calgary, AB, Canada   Robert A. Stebbins

Contents

Chapter 1
Conceptual Background

Abstract The serious leisure perspective is presented in sufficient detail to show how project-based leisure fits in that framework and how PBL relates to well-being. The working definition of leisure is the following: it is un-coerced, contextually framed activity engaged in during free time perceived as such, which people want to do and, using their abilities and resources, actually do in either a satisfying or a fulfilling way, if not both. The SLP forms, in the main, the theoretic foundation for the definitional work reported in this book. Among the general theories typically considered in leisure studies, the SLP is the only one rooted substantially in research on free-time activity. More precisely, the Perspective grew inductively from a foundational set of eight exploratory studies of a sample of leisure activities carried out between 1973 and 1988. Thus the SLP can be described as an *internal* theory and contrasted with the various *external* theories that have also been used to explain this sphere of life.

Keywords Definition of leisure · Serious leisure perspective · Self-fulfillment · Exploratory research · Project-based leisure · Casual leisure · Serious pursuits · Leisure as activity · Leisure as experience · Flow

Project-based leisure (PBL) is one of the three forms comprising the serious leisure perspective (SLP), the other two being the serious pursuits and casual leisure. The goal of this chapter is to present the SLP in sufficient detail to show how PBL fits in that framework and how PBL relates to well-being[1] (the chapter is enlarged from Stebbins (2005) and subsequent publications). Our working definition is the following: leisure is un-coerced, contextually framed activity engaged in during free time perceived as such, which people want to do and, using their abilities and resources, actually do in either a satisfying or a fulfilling way, if not both (Stebbins, 2020).

---

[1] This chapter has appeared in more or less the same form and content in nearly all my monographs on leisure from Stebbins (2004/2014) to the present (n = 22). These works explore one or a few aspects of the SLP, and readers need an in-depth understanding of the Perspective as background for their reading. Referring them to another book for this purpose, is a tortuous route to such learning, when it can be effectively accomplished in an accompanying chapter.

The SLP forms, in the main, the theoretic foundation for the definitional work reported in this book. Among the general theories typically considered in leisure studies, the SLP is the only one rooted substantially in research on free-time activity. More precisely, the Perspective grew inductively from a foundational set of eight exploratory studies of a sample of leisure activities dating from 1973 (summarized in Stebbins, 1992, 2001a, 2007/2015). Thus the SLP can be described as an *internal* theory and contrasted with the various *external* theories that have also been used to explain this sphere of life. Such theories as functionalism, symbolic interactionism, critical analysis, and postmodernism contain certain ideas about leisure, but those ideas emerged with reference to intellectual interests quite distant from leisure. It follows that, when searching for the basic principles with which to create a definition of leisure, whether detailed or condensed, it is best to look for them in this phenomenon's internal theory and research. Here is where we are most likely to discover its essence, its unique features.

Leisure as Activity

Our definition above referred to "un-coerced activity." An *activity* is a type of pursuit, wherein participants in it mentally or physically (often both) think or do something, motivated by the hope of achieving a desired end (Stebbins, 2020). *It is a basic life concept both in the SLP and outside it.* Our existence is filled with activities, both pleasant and unpleasant: sleeping, mowing the lawn, taking the train to work, having a tooth filled, eating lunch, playing tennis matches, running a meeting, and on and on. Activities, as this list illustrates, may be categorized as work, leisure, or non-work obligation. They are, furthermore, general. In some instances, they refer to the behavioral side of recognizable roles, for example commuter, tennis player, and chair of a meeting. In others we may recognize the activity but not conceive of it so formally as a role, exemplified in someone sleeping, mowing a lawn, or eating lunch (not as patron in a restaurant).

The concept of activity is an abstraction, and as such, one broader than that of role. In other words, roles are associated with particular statuses, or positions, in society, whereas with activities, some are status based whereas others are not. For instance, sleeper is not a status, even if sleeping is an activity. It is likewise with lawn mower (person). Sociologists, anthropologists, and psychologists tend to see social relations in terms of roles, and as a result, overlook activities whether aligned with a role or not. Meanwhile certain important parts of life consist of engaging in activities not recognized as roles. Where would many of us be could we not routinely sleep or eat lunch?

Moreover, another dimension distinguishes role and activity, namely, that of statics and dynamics. Roles are static whereas activities are dynamic. Roles, classically conceived of, are relatively inactive expectations for behavior, whereas in activities, people are actually behaving, mentally or physically thinking about or doing something to achieve certain ends. This dynamic quality provides a powerful explanatory link between an activity and a person's desire to participate in it. Nevertheless, the idea of role *is* useful, since participants do encounter role expectations in certain activities (e.g., those in sport, work, volunteering). Although the concept of activity does not include these expectations, in its dynamism, it can, much more effectively than role, account for free-time invention and human agency. In addition, roles and activities, as will become evident in later chapters, are often central points of operation for groups, organizations, social movements, and the like. Finally, both concepts are linchpins linking the social individual to his or her internal psychology, to personality, motivation, attitudes, emotions, and so on.

This definition of activity gets further amplified in the concept of *core activity*: a distinctive set of interrelated actions or steps that must be followed to achieve the outcome or product that a participant seeks. As with general activities core activities are pursued in work, leisure, and non-work obligation. Consider some examples in serious leisure: a core activity of alpine skiing is descending snow-covered slopes, in cabinet making it is shaping and finishing wood, and in volunteer fire fighting is putting out blazes and rescuing people from them. In each case the participant takes several interrelated steps to successfully ski down-hill, make a cabinet, or rescue someone. In casual leisure core activities, which are much less complex than in serious leisure, are exemplified in the actions required to hold sociable conversations with friends, savor beautiful scenery, and offer simple volunteer services (e.g., handing out leaflets, directing traffic in a theater parking lot, clearing snow off the neighborhood hockey rink). Work-related core activities are seen in, for instance, the actions of a surgeon during an operation or the improvisations on a melody by a jazz clarinetist. The core activity in mowing a lawn (as non-work obligation) is pushing or riding the mower. Executing an attractive core activity and its component steps and actions is a main feature drawing participants to the general activity encompassing it, because this core directly enables them to reach a cherished goal. It is the opposite for disagreeable core activities. In short, the core activity has motivational value of its own, even if more strongly held for some activities than others and even if some activities are disagreeable but still must be done.

Core activities can be classified as simple or complex, the two concepts finding their place at opposite poles of a continuum. The location of a core activity on this continuum partially explains its appeal or lack thereof. Most casual leisure is comprised of a set of simple core activities. Here *Homo otiosus* needs only turn on the television set, observe the scenery, drink the glass of wine (no oenophile is he), or gossip about someone. Complexity in casual leisure increases slightly when playing a board game using dice, participating in a Hash House Harrier treasure hunt, or serving as a casual volunteer by, say, collecting bottles for the Scouts or making tea and coffee after a religious service. Additionally, Harrison's (2001) study of upper-middle-class Canadian mass tourists revealed a certain level of complexity in their sensual experience of the touristic sites they visited. For people craving the simple things in life, this is the kind of leisure to head for. The other two domains abound with equivalent simple core activities, as in the work of a restaurant cashier (receiving cash/making change) or the efforts of a householder whose non-work obligation of the day is raking leaves.

So, if complexity is what people want, they must look elsewhere. Leisure projects are necessarily more complex than casual leisure activities. The types of projects covered in this book are, I believe, ample proof of that. Nonetheless, they are not nearly as complex as the core activities around which the serious pursuits revolve. The accumulated knowledge, skill, training, and experience of, for instance, the amateur trumpet player, hobbyist stamp collector, and volunteer emergency medical worker are vast, and defy full description of how they are applied during conduct of the core activity. Of course, neophytes in the serious leisure activities lack these acquisitions, though it is unquestionably their intention to acquire them to a level where they will feel fulfilled. As with simple core activities complex equivalents also exist in the other two domains. Examples in work include the two earlier examples of the surgeon and the jazz clarinetist. In the non-work domain two common examples demonstrate a noticeable level of complexity: driving in city traffic and, for some people, preparing the annual income tax return.

Activity as just defined is, by and large, a foreign idea in psychology, anthropology, and sociology. Sure, scholars there sometimes talk about, for instance, criminal, political, or economic activity, but in so doing, they are referring, in general terms, to a broad category of behavior, not a particular set of actions comprising a pursuit. Instead, our positive concept of activity knows its greatest currency in the interdisciplinary fields of leisure studies and physical education and, more recently, kinesiology. And I suspect that the first adopted the idea from the second. There has always been, in physical education, discussion of and research on activities promoting conditioning, exercise, outdoor interests, human movement, and so on.

Moreover, leisure is positive activity. Positiveness is a personal sentiment felt by existence, rewarding, attractive, and therefore worth living (Seligman & Csikszentmihalyi, 2000; Stebbins, 2009). Such people feel positive about these aspects of life. Because of this sentiment they may also feel positive toward life in general. A primary focus of positive social scientific research is on how, when, where, and why people pursue those things in life that they desire, on the things they do to create a worthwhile existence that, in combination, is substantially rewarding, satisfying, and fulfilling. General and core activities, sometimes joined with role, most of the time agreeable, but some of the time disagreeable, form the cornerstone of separatxesleisure. It is through certain activities that people, propelled by their own agency, find positive things in life, which they blend and balance with certain negative things they must also deal with. Activities, positive and negative, are carried out in the domains of work, leisure, and non-work obligation (Stebbins, 2018, p. 5). Given their institutional nature, these three are best covered in Chap. 7.

Leisure as Experience

The experiential side of leisure (Stebbins, 2012, pp. 10–12) also finds a place in our short definition in the phrase: "activity which people want to do and, in either a satisfying or a fulfilling way (or both) ..." Thus the three basic forms of leisure discussed later in this chapter—casual, serious, and project-based—offer either satisfaction or fulfillment and, at times, both. Some serious leisure, we will see shortly, also offers the experience of psychological flow. In brief, an activity is the means for having a certain leisure experience—*thus when we speak of leisure activity, we speak of its leisure experience, whether satisfying, fulfilling, or both* (Veal, 2016, misses this crucial point—see Stebbins, 2016). The theoretic advantage of linking experience, a psychological state, with activity is that the latter, also being social, has a place in the meso and macro levels of leisure analysis and theory discussed in the following chapters.

Activity, with its experiential component, is a vital linchpin in leisure theory. Driver (2003, p. 168), who stresses the intrinsic nature of leisure behavior, holds that the leisure experience is a cardinal instance of it:

> Given that a human experience is a psychological or physiological response to encountering something, a leisure experience would be any such response to a recreational engagement. All leisure experiences occur at the level of the individual, albeit strongly influenced by social and cultural contexts. Experiences can be psychological, physiological, or psycho-physiological in nature. As with humans, leisure experiences have cognitive, affective, and connotative compounds.

People participating in leisure activities have as a main goal the desire for a satisfying or a fulfilling *core* experience. Furthermore, they evaluate their involvement in these activities as good or bad, according to the level of satisfaction or fulfillment found there.

Flow is arguably the most widely examined generic intrinsic reward in the psychology of work and leisure. Some types of work and leisure generate little or no flow for their participants, whereas those that do can usually be classified either as "devotee occupations" (Stebbins, 2004b) or as serious leisure. Still, it seems that every work and leisure activity capable of generating flow does so in unique fashion. Thus each activity must be closely studied to document the distinctive properties contributing to the kind of flow it offers. I will further elaborate in the next section on the proposition that finding flow is a major source of motivation in some areas of the SLP.

The definition of leisure presented below is intended to bridge the *individual* and *contextual* approaches, with both being equally important in defining leisure. From these two angles leisure is both seen and experienced by the individual participant and seen as implanted in the wider social, cultural, historical, and geographical world. This is the definition of leisure underpinning the SLP.

Serious Leisure Perspective

Only those elements of the SLP are presented here that are needed to understand the place of leisure in PBL. In its most general sense, the Perspective is the conceptual framework that synthesizes three main forms of leisure showing, at once, their distinctive features, similarities, and interrelationships (the SLP is discussed in detail in Stebbins, 2012, 2007/2015, 2020). The Perspective also explains how the three forms—serious pursuits (serious leisure/devotee work), casual leisure, and project-based leisure—are shaped by various psychological, social, cultural, and historical conditions. Each form serves as a conceptual umbrella for a range of types of related activities (see Fig. 1.1). For a brief historical account of the SLP, see the history page at www.seriousleisure.net or, for a longer version, see Stebbins (2020).

Serious leisure is systematic pursuit of an amateur, hobbyist, or volunteer activity that participants find so substantial, interesting, and fulfilling that, in the typical case, they launch themselves on a (leisure) career centered on acquiring and expressing its special skills, knowledge, and experience (Stebbins, 1992, 2001a). The term was coined by the author (Stebbins, 1982) to express the way the people he interviewed and observed viewed the importance of these three kinds of activity in their everyday lives. The adjective "serious" (a word the respondents often used) embodies such qualities as earnestness, sincerity, importance, and carefulness, rather than gravity, solemnity, joylessness, distress, and anxiety. Although the second set of terms occasionally describes serious leisure events, they are uncharacteristic of them and fail to nullify, or, in many cases, even dilute, the overall fulfillment gained by the participants. The idea of "career" in this definition follows sociological tradition, where careers are seen as available in all substantial, complex roles, including those in leisure. Finally, as will be noted shortly, serious leisure is distinct from casual leisure and project-based leisure.

Amateurs are found in art, science, sport, and entertainment, where they are invariably linked in a variety of ways with professional counterparts. The two can be distinguished descriptively in that the activity in question constitutes all or part of a livelihood for professionals but not for amateurs. Furthermore, most professionals work full-time at the activity whereas most amateurs pursue it part-time. The part-time professionals in art and entertainment complicate this picture; although they work part-time, their work is judged by other professionals and by the amateurs as of professional quality. Amateurs and professionals are linked in and therefore defined by a system of relations linking them and their publics—"the P-A-P system" (discussed in more detail in Stebbins 1979, 1992, Chap. 3; Stebbins, 2020, pp. 22–23). Hobbyists lack this professional alter ego, suggesting that, historically, all amateurs were hobbyists before their fields professionalized (see the five types in Fig. 1.1). Both types are drawn to their leisure pursuits significantly more by self-interest than by other-serving altruism, whereas being oriented by the latter, volunteers engage in activities requiring a more or less equal blend of these two motives.

Volunteering is uncoerced help offered either formally or informally with no or, at most, token pay and done for the benefit of both other people (beyond the volunteer's immediate family) and the volunteer (Stebbins, 2015). This conception of volunteering revolves, in significant part, around a central motivational question: it must be determined whether volunteers feel they are engaging in an enjoyable (casual leisure), fulfilling (serious leisure), or enjoyable or fulfilling (project-based leisure) core activity that they have had the option to accept or reject on their own terms. A key element in the leisure conception of volunteering is the felt absence of moral coercion to do the volunteer activity, an element that, in "marginal

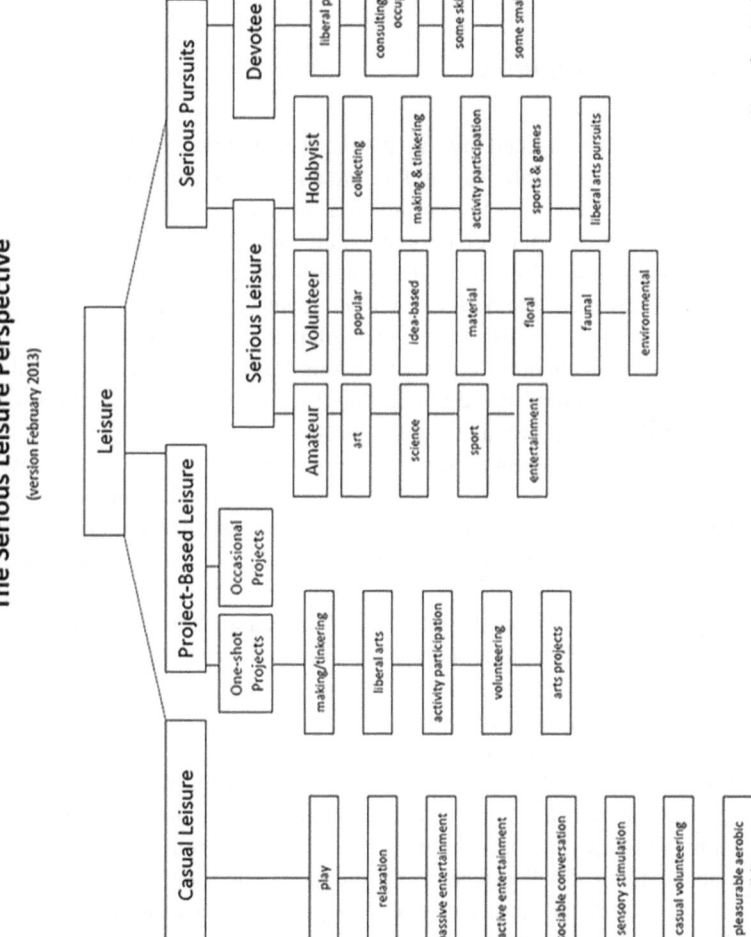

Fig. 1.1 The serious leisure perspective

volunteering" (Stebbins, 2001c) may be experienced in degrees, as more or less coercive.

The reigning conception of volunteering in nonprofit sector research is not that of volunteering as leisure, however, but rather volunteering as unpaid work. The first— an *economic* conception—defines volunteering as the absence of payment as livelihood, whether in money or in kind. This definition, for the most part, leaves unanswered the messy question of motivation so crucial to the second definition, which is a *volitional* conception.

Six Distinguishing Qualities

Serious leisure is further defined by six distinctive qualities, qualities uniformly found among its amateurs, hobbyists, and volunteers. One is the occasional need to *persevere*. Participants who want to continue experiencing the same level of fulfillment in the activity have to meet certain challenges from time to time. Thus, musicians must practice assiduously to master difficult musical passages, baseball players must throw repeatedly to perfect favorite pitches, and volunteers must search their imaginations for new approaches with which to help children with reading problems. It happens in all three types of serious leisure that deepest fulfillment sometimes comes at the end of the activity rather than during it, from sticking with it through thick and thin, from conquering adversity.

Another quality distinguishing all three types of serious leisure is the opportunity to follow a (leisure) *career* in the endeavor, a career shaped by its own special contingencies, turning points, and stages of achievement and involvement. A career that, in some fields, notably certain arts and sports, may nevertheless include decline. Moreover, most, if not all, careers here owe their existence to a third quality: serious leisure participants make significant personal *effort* using their specially acquired knowledge, training, or skill and, indeed at times, all three. Careers for serious leisure participants unfold along lines of their efforts to achieve, for instance, a high level of showmanship, athletic prowess, or scientific knowledge or to accumulate formative experiences in a volunteer role.

Serious leisure is further distinguished by numerous *durable benefits*, or tangible, salutary outcomes of such activity for its participants. They are self-actualization, self-enrichment, self-expression, regeneration or renewal of self, feelings of accomplishment, enhancement of self-image, social interaction and sense of belonging, and lasting physical products of the activity (e.g., a painting, scientific paper, piece of furniture). A further benefit—self-gratification, or pure fun, which is by far the most evanescent benefit in this list—is also enjoyed by casual leisure participants. The possibility of realizing such benefits constitutes a powerful goal in serious leisure.

Fifth, serious leisure is distinguished by a unique *ethos* that emerges in connection with each expression of it. An ethos is the spirit of the community of serious leisure participants, as manifested in shared attitudes, practices, values, beliefs, goals, and so on. The social world of the participants is the organizational milieu in which the associated ethos—at bottom a cultural formation—is expressed (as attitudes, beliefs, values) or realized (as practices, goals). According to Unruh (1980) every social world has its characteristic groups, events, routines, practices, and organizations. It is held together, to an important degree, by semiformal, or mediated, communication. In other words, in the typical case, social worlds are neither heavily bureaucratized nor substantially organized through intense face-to-face interaction. Rather, communication is commonly mediated by newsletters, posted notices, telephone messages, mass mailings, radio and television announcements, and similar means.

The social world is a diffuse, amorphous entity to be sure, but nevertheless one of great importance in the impersonal, segmented life of the modern urban community. Its importance is further amplified by a parallel element of the special ethos, which is missing from Unruh's conception, namely that such worlds are also constituted of a rich subculture. One function of this subculture is to interrelate the many components of this diffuse and amorphous entity. In other words, there is associated with each social world a set of special norms, values, beliefs, styles, moral principles, performance standards, and similar shared representations.

The sixth quality—participants in serious leisure tend to identify strongly with their chosen pursuits—springs from the presence of the other five distinctive qualities. In contrast, most casual leisure, although not usually humiliating or despicable, is nonetheless too fleeting, mundane, and commonplace to become the basis for a distinctive *identity* for most people.

Furthermore, certain rewards and costs come with pursuing a hobbyist, amateur, or volunteer activity. As the following list shows, the rewards are predominantly personal.

Personal Rewards

1. Personal enrichment (cherished experiences)
2. Self-actualization (developing skills, abilities, knowledge)
3. Self-expression (expressing skills, abilities, knowledge already developed)
4. Self-image (known to others as a particular kind of serious leisure participant)
5. Self-gratification (combination of superficial enjoyment and deep satisfaction)
6. Re-creation (regeneration) of oneself through serious leisure after a day's work
7. Financial return (from a serious leisure activity)

Social Rewards

8. Social attraction (associating with other serious leisure participants, with clients as a volunteer, participating in the social world of the activity)
9. Group accomplishment (group effort in accomplishing a serious leisure project; senses of helping, being needed, being altruistic)
10. Contribution to the maintenance and development of the group (including senses of helping, being needed, being altruistic in making the contribution)

Further, every serious leisure activity contains its own costs—a distinctive combination of tensions, dislikes and disappointments—which each participant confronts in his or her own way. Tensions and dislikes develop within the activity or through its imperfect mesh with work, family, and other leisure interests. Put more precisely, the goal of gaining fulfillment in serious leisure is the drive to experience the rewards of a given leisure activity, such that its costs are seen by the participant as more or less insignificant by comparison. This is at once the meaning of the activity for the participant and that person's motivation for engaging in it. It is this motivational sense of the concept of reward that distinguishes it from the idea of durable benefit set out earlier, an idea that emphasizes outcomes rather than antecedent conditions. Nonetheless, the two ideas constitute two sides of the same social psychological coin.

Devotee Work

In Stebbins (2012) I joined serious leisure and devotee work under the heading of the *serious pursuits*, which now bridge its two types. The present section explains this classificatory change, from what was to this point in the history of the SLP a separation of the two as leisure and work, respectively. The justification for this change is simple: devotee work is essentially leisure. So we should call this spade a spade and explore it as part of the Perspective.

Occupational devotees feel a powerful devotion, or strong, positive attachment, to a form of self-enhancing work. In such work the sense of achievement is high and the core activity endowed with such intense appeal that the line between this work and leisure is virtually erased (Stebbins, 2004b, 2022). Further, it is by way of the core activity of their work that devotees realize a unique combination of, what are for them, strongly seated cultural values (Williams Jr., 2000, p. 146): success, achievement, freedom of action, individual personality, and activity (being involved in something meaningful). Other categories of workers may also be animated by some, even all, of these values, but fail for various reasons to realize them in gainful employment.

Occupational devotees turn up chiefly, though not exclusively, in four areas of the economy, providing their work there is, at most, only lightly bureaucratized: certain small businesses, the skilled trades, the consulting and counseling occupations, and the public- and client-centered professions. Public-centered professions are found in the arts, sports, scientific, and entertainment fields, while those that are client-centered abound in such fields as law, teaching, accounting, and medicine (Stebbins, 1992, p. 22). It is assumed in all this that the work and its core activity to which people become devoted carries with it a respectable personal and social identity within their reference groups, since it would be difficult, if not impossible, to be devoted to work that those groups regarded with scorn. Still, positive identification with the job is not a defining condition of occupational devotion, since such identification can develop for other reasons, including high salary, prestigious employer, and advanced educational qualifications.

The fact of devotee work for some people and its possibility for others signals that work, as one of life's domains, can be highly positive. Granted, most workers are not fortunate enough to find such work. For those who do find it, however, the work meets six criteria (Stebbins, 2004b, p. 9). To generate occupational devotion:

1. the valued core activity must be profound; to perform it acceptability requires substantial skill, knowledge, or experience or a combination of two or three of these;
2. the core must offer significant variety;
3. the core must also offer significant opportunity for creative or innovative work, as a valued expression of individual personality. The adjectives 'creative' and 'innovative' stress that the undertaking results in something new or different, showing imagination and application of routine skill or knowledge. That is, boredom is likely to develop only after the onset of fatigue experienced from long hours on the job, a point at which significant creativity and innovation are no longer possible;
4. the would-be devotee must have reasonable control over the amount and disposition of time put into the occupation (the value of freedom of action), such that he can prevent it from becoming a burden. Medium and large bureaucracies have tended to subvert this criterion. For, in interest of the survival and development of their organization, managers have felt they must deny their nonunionized employees this freedom, and force them to accept stiff deadlines and heavy workloads. But no activity, be it leisure or work, is so appealing that it invites unlimited participation during all waking hours;
5. the would-be devotee must have both an aptitude and a taste for the work in question. This is, in part, a case of one man's meat being another man's poison. John finds great fulfillment in being a physician, an occupation that holds little appeal for Jane who, instead, adores being a lawyer (work John finds unappealing);
6. the devotees must work in a physical and social milieu that encourages them to pursue often and without significant constraint the core activity. This includes avoidance of excessive paperwork, caseloads, class sizes, market demands, and the like.

Sounds ideal, if not idealistic, but in fact occupations and work roles exist that meet these criteria. In today's climate of occupational deskilling, over-bureaucratization, and similar impediments to fulfilling core activity at work, many people find it difficult to locate or arrange devotee employment. The six criteria just listed also characterize serious leisure, giving further substance to the claim put forward here that such leisure and devotee work occupy a great deal of common ground. Together they constitute the class of serious pursuits.

Casual Leisure

Casual leisure is immediately intrinsically rewarding, relatively short-lived pleasurable activity requiring little or no special training to enjoy it. It is fundamentally hedonic, pursued for its significant level of pure enjoyment, or pleasure. The termed was coined by the author in the 1982a conceptual statement about serious leisure, which at the time, depicted its casual counterpart as all activity not classifiable as serious (project-based leisure has since been added as a third form, see next section). As a scientific concept casual leisure languished in this residual status, until Stebbins (1997, 2001a), belatedly recognizing its centrality and importance in leisure studies, sought to elaborate the idea as a sensitizing concept for exploratory research, as he had earlier for serious leisure (see also Rojek, 1997). It is considerably less substantial and offers no career of the sort found in serious leisure.

Its types—there are eight—include *play* (including dabbling), relaxation (e.g., sitting, napping, strolling), *passive entertainment* (e.g., TV, books, recorded music), *active entertainment* (e.g., games of chance, party games), *sociable conversation*, *sensory stimulation* (e.g., sex, eating, drinking), and *casual volunteering* (as opposed to serious leisure, or career, volunteering). The last and newest type—*pleasurable aerobic activity*—refers to physical activities that require effort sufficient to cause marked increase in respiration and heart rate.

Here I am referring to "aerobic activity" in the broad sense, to all activity that calls for such effort, which to be sure, includes the routines pursued collectively in (narrowly conceived of) aerobics classes and those pursued individually by way of televised or video-taped programs of aerobics (Stebbins, 2004a). Yet, as with its passive and active cousins in entertainment, pleasurable aerobic activity is basically casual leisure. That is, to do such activity requires little more than minimal skill, knowledge, or experience. Examples include the game of the Hash House Harriers (a type of treasure hunt in the outdoors), kickball (described in *The Economist* 2005, as a cross between soccer and baseball), and such children's games as hide-and-seek.

It is likely that people pursue the different types of casual leisure in combinations of two and three at least as often as they pursue them separately. For instance, every type can be relaxing, producing in this fashion play-relaxation, passive entertainment-relaxation, and so on. Various combinations of play and sensory stimulation are also possible, as in experimenting with drug use, sexual activity, and thrill seeking in movement. Additionally, sociable conversation accompanies some sessions of sensory stimulation (e.g., recreational drug use, curiosity seeking, displays of beauty) as well as some sessions of relaxation and active and passive entertainment, although such conversation normally tends to be rather truncated in the latter two.

Notwithstanding its hedonic nature casual leisure is by no means wholly frivolous, for some clear costs and benefits accrue from pursuing it. Moreover, in contrast to the evanescent hedonic property of casual leisure itself, these costs and benefits are enduring. The benefits include serendipitous creativity and discovery in play, regeneration from early intense activity, and development and maintenance of interpersonal relationships (Stebbins, 2001b). Some of its costs root in excessive casual leisure or lack of variety as manifested in boredom or lack of time for leisure activities that contribute to self through acquisition of skills, knowledge, and experience (i.e., serious leisure). Moreover, casual leisure is alone unlikely to produce a distinctive leisure identity.

Project-Based Leisure

Project-based leisure (Stebbins, 2005)—a third form of leisure activity—requires considerable planning, effort, and sometimes skill or knowledge, but is for all that neither serious leisure nor intended to develop into such. Examples include such time-limited undertakings as surprise birthday parties, elaborate preparations for a major holiday, and volunteering for sports events. Though only a rudimentary social world springs up around the project, it does in its own particular way bring together friends, neighbors, or relatives (e.g., drawn by a genealogical project or Christmas celebrations), or pull the individual participant into an organizational milieu (e.g., through volunteering for a sports event or major convention).

Types of Project-Based Leisure

Leisure projects cannot logically be part of a lifestyle, since they are undertaken irregularly. The concept will nonetheless be discussed, because it plays a complementary role in understanding how our leisure lifestyles are enacted. It was noted in the definition just presented that project-based leisure is not all the same. Whereas systematic exploration may reveal others, two types are presently evident: one-shot projects and occasional projects. These are presented next using the earlier classificatory framework for amateur, hobbyist, and volunteer activities developed by the author (see also Fig. 1.1).

One-Shot Projects

In all these projects people generally use the talents and knowledge they have at hand, even though for some projects they may seek certain instructions beforehand, including reading a book or taking a short course. And some projects resembling hobbyist activity participation may require a modicum of preliminary conditioning. Always, the goal is to undertake successfully the one-shot project and nothing more, and sometimes a small amount of background preparation is necessary for this. It is possible that a survey would show that most project-based leisure is hobbyist in character and the next most common, a kind of volunteering. First, the following hobbyist-like projects have so far been identified:

- Making and tinkering:
  - Interlacing, interlocking, and knot-making from kits
  - Other kit assembly projects (e.g., stereo tuner, craft store projects)
  - Do-it-yourself projects done primarily for fulfillment, some of which may even be undertaken with minimal skill and knowledge (e.g., build a rock wall or a fence, finish a room in the basement, plant a special garden). This could turn into an irregular series of such projects, spread over many years, possibly even transforming the participant into a hobbyist.

- Liberal arts:
  - Genealogy (not as ongoing hobby)
  - Tourism: special trip, not as part of an extensive personal tour program, to visit different parts of a region, a continent, or much of the world

- Activity participation: long back-packing trip, canoe trip; one-shot mountain ascent (e.g., Fuji, Rainier, Kilimanjaro)

One-shot volunteering projects are also common, though possibly somewhat less so than hobbyist-like projects. And less common than either are the amateur-like projects, which seem to concentrate in the sphere of theater.

- Volunteering
  - Volunteer at a convention or conference, whether local, national, or international in scope.
  - Volunteer at a sporting competition, whether local, national, or international in scope.
  - Volunteer at an arts festival or special exhibition mounted in a museum.
  - Volunteer to help restore human life or wildlife after a natural or human-made disaster caused by, for instance, a hurricane, earthquake, oil spill, or industrial accident.

- Arts projects:
  - Entertainment theatre: produce a skit or one-off community pageant; prepare a home film, video or set of photos.
  - Public speaking: prepare a talk for a reunion, an after-dinner speech, an oral position statement on an issue to be discussed at a community meeting.
  - Memoirs: therapeutic audio, visual and written productions by the elderly; life histories and autobiographies (all ages); accounts of personal events (all ages) (Stebbins, 2011).

Occasional Projects

The occasional projects seem more likely to originate in or be motivated by an agreeable obligation than their one-shot cousins. Examples of occasional projects include the sum of the culinary, decorative, or other creative activities undertaken, for example, at home or at work for a religious occasion or someone's birthday. Likewise, national holidays and similar celebrations sometimes inspire individuals to mount occasional projects consisting of an ensemble of inventive elements.

Unlike one-shot projects occasional projects have the potential to become routinized, which happens when new creative possibilities no longer come to mind as the participant arrives at a fulfilling formula wanting no further modification. North Americans who decorate their homes the same way each Christmas season exemplify this situation. Indeed, it can happen that, over the years, such projects may lose their appeal, but not their necessity, thereby becoming disagreeable obligations, which their authors no longer define as leisure.

And, lest it be overlooked, note that one-shot projects also hold the possibility of becoming unpleasant. Thus, the hobbyist genealogist gets overwhelmed with the details of family history and the difficulty of verifying dates. The thought of putting in time and effort doing something once considered leisure, but which she now dislikes, makes no sense. Likewise, volunteering for a project may turn sour, creating in the volunteer a sense of being faced with a disagreeable obligation, which however, must nonetheless be honored. This is leisure no more.

Conclusions

The SLP attempts to embrace all leisure activity worldwide. This lofty goal is a long way from being met at present, given the paucity of research on leisure in its name, especially in non-Western societies, and in the modern rapid emergence of new leisure across the planet. Still, the SLP does show how PBL and well-being fit in the use of free time, as the following chapters attest. We start with projects regarded by participants as opportune ways of passing interstitial time.

References

Driver, B. (2003). Benefits. In J. M. Jenkins & J. J. Pigram (Eds.), *Encyclopedia of leisure and outdoor recreation* (pp. 31–36). Routledge.

Harrison, J. (2001). Thinking about tourists. *International Sociology, 16,* 159–172.

Rojek, C. (1997). Leisure theory: Retrospect and prospect. *Loisir et Société/Society and Leisure, 20,* 383–400.

Seligman, M. E. P., & Csikszentmihalyi, M. (2000). Positive psychology: An introduction. *American Psychologist, 55*(1), 5–14.

Stebbins, R. A. (1979). *Amateurs: On the margin between work and leisure.* Sage.

Stebbins, R. A. (1982). Serious leisure: A conceptual statement. *Pacific Sociological Review, 25,* 251–272.

Stebbins, R. A. (1992). *Amateurs, professionals, and serious leisure.* McGill- Queen's University Press.

Stebbins, R. A. (1997). Casual leisure: A conceptual statement. *Leisure Studies, 16,* 17–25.

Stebbins, R. A. (2001a). *New directions in the theory and research of serious leisure* (Mellen studies in sociology) (Vol. 28). Edwin Mellen.

Stebbins, R. A. (2001b). The costs and benefits of hedonism: Some consequences of taking casual leisure seriously. *Leisure Studies, 20*, 305–309.

Stebbins, R. A. (2001c). Volunteering – Mainstream and marginal: Preserving the leisure experience. In M. Graham & M. Foley (Eds.), *Volunteering in leisure: Marginal or inclusive?* (Vol. 75, pp. 1–10). Leisure Studies Association.

Stebbins, R. A. (2004a). Pleasurable aerobic activity: A type of casual leisure with salubrious implications. *World Leisure Journal, 46*(4), 55–58.

Stebbins, R. A. (2004b). *Between work and leisure: The common ground of two separate worlds.* New Brunswick/New York: Transaction/Routledge, 2017. (Paperback edition with new Preface, 2014).

Stebbins, R. A. (2005). Project-based leisure: Theoretical neglect of a common use of free time. *Leisure Studies, 24*, 1–11.

Stebbins, R. A. (2007/2015). *Serious leisure: A perspective for our time.* New Brunswick/New York: Transaction/Routledge, 2017. (Published in paperback in 2015 with new Preface).

Stebbins, R. A. (2009). *Personal decisions in the public square: Beyond problem solving into a positive sociology.* Transaction.

Stebbins, R. A. (2011). Personal memoirs, project-based leisure and therapeutic recreation for seniors. *Leisure Reflections*, no. 26 in *LSA Newsletter*, no. 88, March, pp. 29–31. Also available in www.seriousleisure.net/Digital library.

Stebbins, R. A. (2012). *The idea of leisure: First principles.* Transaction.

Stebbins, R. A. (2015). *Leisure and the motive to volunteer: Theories of serious, casual, and project-based leisure.* Palgrave Macmillan.

Stebbins, R. A. (2016). *The serious leisure perspective or the leisure experience perspective? A rejoinder to Veal.* Published in Research Gate, https://doi.org/10.13140/RG.2.2.31471.23203.

Stebbins, R. A. (2018). *Social worlds and the leisure experience.* Bingley.

Stebbins, R. A. (2020). *The serious leisure perspective: A Synthesis.* Palgrave Macmillan.

Stebbins, R. A. (2022). *Occupational devotion: Finding satisfaction and fulfillment at work.* Anthem Press.

Unruh, D. R. (1980). The nature of social worlds. *Pacific Sociological Review, 23*, 271–296.

Veal, A. J. (2016). The serious leisure perspective and the experience of leisure. *Leisure Sciences.* doi:https://doi.org/10.1080/01490400.2016.1189367.

Williams, R. M., Jr. (2000). American society. In E. F. Borgatta & R. J. V. Montgomery (Eds.), *Encyclopedia of sociology* (Vol. 1, 2nd ed., pp. 140–148). Macmillan.

Chapter 2
Opportune Activities

Abstract This chapter offers the broadest canvas portraying PBL found in this book as such leisure bears on subjective well-being. The following subjects are covered: PBL as intriguing activity, as consisting of making things, as liberal arts activities, as activity participation, as artistic expression, and as one-off volunteering. The PBL activities are considered interstitial, and their meaning to the individual is anchored in this understanding of them, as is their signal capacity for generating that person's well-being. Apart from these conditions most of the activities considered here are of interest to the participant, in the sense that they are domestic or, if outside the home, are easily accessible. Given this quality they can in effect serve interstitially as time fillers. Most are also reasonably inexpensive. This said, certain activities are treated of as resembling a liberal art or a participant activity that do encourage some people to travel far from home.

Keywords Intriguing activity · Well-being · Interstitial activity · Making things · Liberal arts activities · Activity participation · Arts projects · One-off volunteering · Occasional volunteering

This chapter offers the broadest canvas portraying PBL in this book as such leisure bears on subjective well-being. The PBL activities are considered interstitial, and their meaning to the individual is anchored in this understanding of them, as is their signal capacity for generating that person's well-being. Apart from these conditions the activities chosen are immensely varied, depending on among other factors time available, appeal, resources, and approval by intimates.

Most of the activities considered here are of interest to the participant, in the sense that they are domestic or, if outside the home, are easily accessible. Given this quality they can in effect serve interstitially as time fillers. Most are also reasonably inexpensive. This said, I will discuss certain activities treated of as resembling a liberal art or a participant activity that do encourage some people to travel far from home.

Intriguing Activities

Some of the intriguing, mentally-absorbing, PBL activities can often be pursued in two or three hours; they are thus quintessentially interstitial. Evenings after a day's work and a meal is one common period for this kind of leisure. It includes the smaller crossword puzzles and jigsaw puzzles, an issue of a magazine or a chapter or two in a book, or a session of solitaire. To the extent that a person's time available for PBL is normally constrained, meatier projects must therefore be tackled in installments—filling in two or more interstices—as in making a quilt, knitting a sweater, or completing a scrapbook project.

Because they are non-competitive, the puzzles and mazes designed for leisure are not games in the strictest sense of the definition set out below. More accurately, puzzles and mazes are diversions designed to test the ingenuity, knowledge, or insight of the player. The crossword, acrostic, jigsaw, and mechanical puzzles (e.g., Rubik's Cube) are popular, as are the "brain twisters" like hidden pictures, memory tests, and the mathematical and logical puzzles. They make for interesting leisure for people so inclined and fit well as an evening's free-time project.

The puzzles and mazes are neither sports nor games, the latter being inherently competitive activities involving other people. The sports are based on one or more physical skills, which are nonetheless absent in other competitive games. Further, chance figures heavily in many non-sport games, seen in drawing cards, shaking dice, spinning dials and wheels, and so on. Granted, there are also chance elements in sport games, but they are not an inherent part of the game itself. In this sense the non-sport games of chess and checkers resemble sport games.

Since they can never qualify as serious leisure nor as PBL, casual leisure games based purely on chance (e.g., craps, bingo, roulette) are omitted from this discussion. To qualify as serious leisure an activity must make use of developed skills, knowledge, or experience or a combination of these three. A game can have chance components and still become a hobby, however, because it also allows decision-making informed by accumulated knowledge of and experience with the game. Furthermore, games of this sort seem rarely to be played as interstitial projects, though they might be played as exploratory projects, that is, to see if they would make a good hobby or a good casual leisure activity.

Some other casual leisure activities can also be understood as PBL. The breathtaking carnival rides found at amusement parks and theme parks—the oldest being the roller coaster—are a main instance of such leisure projects. The bungee jump is another. At least this proposition holds for participants curious to experience them for the first time.

Finally, initial voluntary experiences with alcohol and recreational drugs can be conceived of in PBL terms, as casual leisure of the sensory stimulation variety. What is it like to be mildly intoxicated with liquor or high on a hallucinogenic drug? The latter can produce changes in a person's state of consciousness seen in major alterations in thought, mood, and perception? The first session with these sensations may not turn out as hoped for, possibly leading to a second experiential project with the same substance (often as inspired by peers).

Thus, a "bad trip" will wind up for some curious souls in search of an agreeable experience as a negative instance of what was to be PBL.

A **bad trip** (also known as **challenging experiences**, **acute intoxication from hallucinogens**, **psychedelic crisis**, or **emergence phenomenon**) is an acute adverse psychological reaction to classic hallucinogens. With proper screening, preparation, and support in a regulated setting these are usually benign. A bad trip on psilocybin, for instance, often features intense anxiety, confusion, and agitation, or even psychotic episodes. As of 2011, exact data on the frequency of bad trips are not available.

Bad trips can be exacerbated by the inexperience or irresponsibility of the user or the lack of proper preparation and environment for the trip, and are often reflective of unresolved psychological tensions triggered during the course of the experience. (*Wikipedia*, "Bad Trips").

Making Things

Leisure projects consisting of making something can take more than 2 or 3 h to complete. Large jigsaw puzzles are an example. According to *Wikipedia* ("Jigsaw Puzzles"), they can take days to complete, sometimes involving a team of participants to accomplish this. Finding the space for such an undertaking can be a challenge as well, especially when the finished puzzle is larger than a standard dining room or ping pong table. The *Wikipedia* site describes some of the large, commercially available puzzles that cover between 15,000 and 17,000 m^2.

These often take days to complete, suggesting that projects of this size and complexity are rarely PBL, but rather the province of serious leisure hobbyists who regularly work on puzzles and even enter contests. Some of them join the World Jigsaw Puzzle Federation, it being made up of associations and fans from more than 50 countries (https://www.worldjigsawpuzzle.org). Working on jigsaw puzzles as well as tabletop games, video games, word and number puzzles, crosswords, Sudoku, and memory games is said to augment the well-being of patients with Altzheimer's disease accomplished by challenging their brains (Altzheimer Society of Canada, https://alzheimer.ca/en).

Quilting is a hobby for most people interested in pursuing it (Stalp, 2007). Still, there are times when one quilted item is all that is wanted, as in a wall hanging or a bedspread for a child. Such one-off projects are possible to execute using a commercial kit (available with instructions) on, for example, Amazon.com). People quilt as PBL items like rainbow keychains, unicorns, headbands, pom poms, mittens, and more. They do this sporadically for themselves, friends, and relatives, as a special way of bonding with them. Small knitting and crocheting projects are additional possibilities (Court, 2020).

Kit assembly is another genre of PBL, one-off activity for adults and teenagers. Models of vehicles, buildings, boats, and cityscapes are common among the offerings on Amazon.com or in hobby/craft shops. Wood carving can be part of such

PBL, especially when packaged as a kit, which includes a whittling knife and wood blocks. Some of the objects carved can be completed in an evening. The same can be said for simple macramé and other interlocking, interlacing, and knot-making projects, as created from kits. See sarahmaker.com (https://sarahmaker.com/craft-kits-for-adults) for a description of 21 crafts (as July 2022) that can be made from kits that amount to PBL as a one-off, interesting activity. As Sarah Stearns observes any one of these projects can, however, generate enough passion to turn into a lasting hobby.

Some domestic do-it-yourself projects are done primarily for short-term fulfillment. And many of them may even be undertaken with minimal skill and knowledge (e.g., build a rock wall or a fence, finish a room in the basement, plant a special garden). Interior and exterior painting projects can fall into this class of leisure. Moreover, these could turn into an irregular series of such projects, spread over many years, possibly even transforming the participant into a hobbyist. Chelsea and Morgan Faulkner provide a list of 50 DIY domestic projects that conform to the definition of PBL (https://www.hgtv.com/how-to/home-improvement/diy-home-projects-pictures). Examples include Paint the Front Door, Install a Shiplap Accent Wall, Set the Mood with String Lights, and Stencil Your Patio.

Creating a family genealogy is a growing leisure interest, at least in Western societies. According to. Genealogy.com, LLC, constructing one's family tree has enjoyed a recent efflorescence, as suggested by a poll carried out in May 2000 by Maritz Marketing Research (*Wikipedia*: Genealogy.Com, retrieved 6 August 2022). The digitization of records, growth of the Internet, desire to locate oneself in the mass of humankind, among other antecedents, help account for this leisure trend (Hershkovitz & Hardof-Jaffe, 2017; Roued et al., 2023).

Making personal histories may begin as PBL: family histories, scrapbooking, and memory journaling or diary writing. Writing a family history, usually the activity of an individual member, often begins as a chronicle of a particular event, such as a significant death, noteworthy honor, divorce, marriage, debilitating accident, or major legal success or failure. In the eyes of the individual, the death, honor, and the like is so momentous that it merits a written account. Furthermore, any of these could be the subject of a scrapbooking project, and some marriages and divorces may be written up as a personal history.

Some personal histories are presented in the form of memoirs. They can be therapeutic audio, visual, or written productions by the elderly containing material bearing on the individual's struggles with certain mental, social, or physical problems. Alternatively, as PBL, some people write life histories of themselves (autobiographies) or close family or friends or they write accounts of important personal events of self or significant others, such as an accident, debilitating disease, or major setback or success at work.

> Personal History helps you—as an individual, family, community, organization, or business—preserve your history through interviews, conversations, or editing your own words. Think heirloom book, paperback, chapbook, radio diary or other audio account, personal memoir, family tribute, annotated photo album or cookbook, letter series, community history, business chronicle, ethical will … there are so many options—let's talk! (source: http://www.personalhistory.org)

As an option, the personal historian might prefer to record the entire event in diary form. As PBL this would require additions to the diary until the event had ended, whether it lasted a few hours, a few days, or much longer. Segal (2022) observes that "writers have long used diaries to make sense of life. Now, diaries can be shared in real time, helping shape public perception of events as they unfold—including war." Thus making a personal history may contain the possibility that the activity may be appealing enough to develop into a hobby, as a long-term pursuit. This is most likely with serious accidents, deaths of significant others, outcomes of protracted legal proceedings, lengthy wars, and so on.

Liberal Arts Activities

The term "liberal arts" appears to be a Western invention, referring as it does to such academic subjects as literature, philosophy, mathematics, and the social and physical sciences. They are seen as distinct from professional and technical subjects such as engineering, medicine, and public administration. Additionally, the concept of liberal arts includes the fine arts, which when the first are studied as leisure projects, are treated of separately as amateur-like pastimes (see below in this chapter and Chap. 4).

The liberal arts activities have been conceptualized as hobbies (Stebbins, 1994). These serious leisure participants are enamored of the systematic acquisition of knowledge for its own sake. Many of them accomplish this by reading voraciously in a field of art, sport, cuisine, language (e.g., Bendle & Pooley, 2016) culture, history, science, philosophy, politics, or literature. Additionally, tourism, video documentaries, and special television programs can also be sources of such knowledge. By contrast, the rest of the serious leisure perspective is mostly anchored in knowledge as a means to carrying out the amateur, hobbyist, or volunteer activity to which the participant is devoted.

The one-off cultural tour fits well in the liberal arts class of PBL. For the person who has longed to do so, a one-time visit to Paris, Scandinavia, South Africa, or Australia is a leisure project often lasting 10 days to 2 weeks (e.g., Palso, 2008). Of much longer duration but PBL nevertheless are the diverse reading and learning projects. One might, for example, decide to read all the winners of the Nobel Prize for Literature of a given year. Or read all the works of a famous novelist. Watching educational documentary films might also be classified as a liberal arts-like interstitial activity, in that some of them can be viewed in a couple of hours (e.g., Michael Moore's *Sicko* and *Fahrenheit 11/9*). Promoting sustainable food and food citizenship through an adult education leisure experience offers its own one-off cultural tour (Warner et al., 2014).

Attending a rally or a march centered on a political or social issue is, as a leisure activity, another facet of this kind of PBL. Here the typical participant is not a volunteer but rather someone interested in acquiring knowledge of the liberal arts variety on the cause of interest. That person's initial presence at such an event is PBL, so long as it is not part of an ongoing liberal arts hobby or volunteer activity (in politics).

Activity Participation

Activity participants constitute a type of hobbyist, enthusiasts who go in for non-competitive, rule-based, pursuits such as fishing, orienteering, and a cappella singing. As PBL such activities are one-off involvements, however, exemplified by a long backpacking or canoe trip or a one-off mountain ascent (e.g., Fuji, Rainier, Kilimanjaro). They generate memorable experiences and the vivid positive expectations of having them prior to departing on the adventure.

A major subcategory of activity participation has been labelled *Nature Activities* (Davidson & Stebbins, 2011). Some of them are *nature appreciation*: hiking, horseback riding, backpacking/wilderness camping, cave exploration (spelunking), bird watching, canoeing, scuba/snorkeling, snowshoeing, and snowmobiling. Any of these can be pursued at a minimal level of competence as one-off PBL, following on some preliminary instruction. The 107-day canoe trip made by a family of four through the western Northwest Territories of Canada constitutes a vivid example of PBL as nature appreciation (Strong, 2022).

Other kinds of nature activity require significant preliminary instruction. This class—*nature challenges*—includes ballooning, wave surfing, alpine skiing, sailing, mountain climbing, and dirt (trail) bike riding. It is likewise for the activities leading to *nature exploitation*, mainly hunting, fishing, trapping, and mushroom picking (Fine, 1998; Presser & Taylor, 2011; Bellenger, 2017). Considerable time must be invested in learning these hobbies to the point where they are satisfying and suggestive of how fulfilling they can become if pursued further. Thus it often happens that the participant continues with such leisure after the first experience with it. These enthusiasts then become neophytes whose mission is to explore the benefits possible in a routine pursuit of the hobby, even if some of them decide in the short run to abandon this budding interest (Stebbins, 2014, pp. 31–32).

Arts Projects

One set of these projects can be labelled entertainment theatre. For instance, it may qualify as PBL when someone mounts a short skit for a special family or community occasion. Also found in this category is creating and showing a home video or set of photos of, for example, one's holiday abroad, a wedding, or a child's birthday party.

Another kind of PBL arts project is the singular public speaking event. Thus, the participant may have to prepare and present a talk for a school reunion, an after-dinner speech, or an oral statement of position on an issue to be discussed at a community meeting. The latter may not always be conceivable as leisure, however, being defined instead as a disagreeable but necessary (nonwork) obligation. Attending some of these events can be seen as PBL, for instance, enjoying a comedy festival (Frew, 2006) or another one-off artistic presentation (e.g., Rossetti & Quinn, 2023).

Are the other arts given to PBL, such as those expressed through music, literature, painting, and dance? We might list here such events as poetry readings, music and dance recitals, and gallery-based exhibitions of a sample of a visual artist's works. Still, to become good enough to participate in these displays of excellence, requires years of amateur development in the art in question. This is not the truncated expressive space of PBL.

Turning to one-off volunteering projects, note that they are also common, though possibly somewhat less so than hobbyist-like projects. Volunteering in major sports competitions (e.g., the Olympic Games, World Cup in rugby), large-scale industrial and academic conferences, and national and international arts festivals are typically one-off activities (see next section). And less common than these volunteer projects are the amateur-like projects, which seem to be pursued mainly in the realm of theater (exemplified by the Fringe Festivals and Wichmann's (2017) study of gymnastics and the exhibition known as the World Gymnaestrada).

One-Off Volunteering as PBL

Volunteering at a convention, conference, or similar gathering, whether local, national, or international in scope, is typically a one-off leisure experience. These events are commonly rotated among a slate of communities such that all members occasionally have a reasonably geographically close opportunity to participate in them. The conventions and conferences are usually sponsored by non-profit associations, whose need for volunteers is well-known, especially local ones who are in the best position to help run these undertakings.

As another example, consider volunteering at a sporting competition, whether local, national, or international in scope. Possibly the archetypical PBL in this area is found in the volunteering activities available for local residents when the Olympic Games come to town. Nevertheless, competitions of lesser prominence sometimes need similar volunteer service, thereby setting up project opportunities in communities that may over the years host those competitions again (e.g., Twynam et al., 2002/2003; Gravelle & Larocque, 2005; Undlien, 2019). They can also offer opportunities for occasional PBL (discussed below).

Volunteering at an arts festival or special exhibition mounted in, say, a museum mostly draws participants seeking a PBL experience. Festivals featuring jazz, crafts, local culture, and the theater arts (e.g., the Fringe Festivals), among others, rely heavily on one-off volunteer help. It is likewise for special events and exhibitions occasionally staged at galleries, museums, and heritage sites (Wensing, 2020).

Volunteering to help restore human life or wildlife after a natural or human-made disaster caused by, for instance, a hurricane, earthquake, oil spill, or industrial accident is commonly a one-off activity. This is likely to demand a long-term commitment by the participant, since the physical damage caused by the event is usually extensive. In the literature on volunteering and nonprofit associations, this kind of leisure has been dubbed "spontaneous volunteering" (Aguirre et al., 2016). Voluntourism may also be conceived of as PBL (see Chen et al., 2018).

Occasional Projects

The occasional projects seem more likely to originate in or be motivated by agreeable obligation than their one-off cousins. Examples of occasional projects include the sum of the culinary, decorative, or other creative activities undertaken, for example, at home or at work for a religious occasion or someone's birthday. Likewise, national holidays and similar celebrations sometimes inspire individuals to mount occasional projects consisting of an ensemble of inventive elements.

Unlike one-off projects occasional projects have the potential to become routinized, which often happens when new creative possibilities no longer come to mind as the participant arrives at a fulfilling formula wanting no further modification. North Americans who decorate their homes the same way each Christmas season exemplify this situation. Indeed, it can happen over the years that these projects lose their appeal, but not their necessity. As such they turn into disagreeable obligations, with their authors no longer defining them as leisure (see, for example, Bella, 1992).

New Vision Psychology (https://newvisionpsychology.com.au/general-counsel ling/christmas-anxiety-is-real-and-this-is-what-you-can-do-about-it/, retrieved 11 November 2022) lists some common stressors and pressures that can be seen as undermining the PBL typically associated with Christmas.

Environmental stressors—examples include:

- Feeling rushed and out of time with having to attend numerous social engagements.
- Tidying up work tasks before the holidays.
- Buying gifts in busy shopping centres.
- Planning events for Christmas and New Years.

Financial stressors—examples include:

- Pressure on tight budgets due to buying gifts, attending social events and holiday activities.
- Restricted income due to days off work.

Relationship pressures—examples include:

- Being obliged (in some cases) to spend time with family members that you would normally try to avoid
- Feeling like your partner is not doing any 'heavy lifting' when it comes to Christmas preparations.

Conclusion

This chapter has centered on activities, many of which can enhance well-being during periods of forced isolation driven by a pandemic, imprisonment, debilitating disease, or severe natural event (e.g., storm, heat wave), to mention a few possibilities. Viewed as interstitial leisure PBL helps the participant construct an optimal leisure lifestyle and the well-being it brings, achieved by eliminating unpleasant gaps of boredom during free time. Finally, PBL can trigger an unwitting sampling of the world of interstitial leisure to discover, however inadvertently, possible serious leisure. Thus, a casual interest in crossword puzzles could bring a puzzler into contact with competitions in this field, transforming that person into a hobbyist by way of regular participation.

Project-based leisure is often pursued under the heading of meeting an agreeable obligation, which is the subject of the next chapter.

References

Aguirre, B. G., Macias-Madrano, J., et al. (2016). Spontaneous volunteering in emergencies. In D. H. Smith, R. A. Stebbins, & J. Grotz (Eds.), *The Palgrave handbook of volunteering, civic participation, and nonprofit associations* (pp. 311–329). Palgrave Macmillan.

Bella, L. (1992). *The Christmas imperative: Leisure, family, and women's work.* Fernwood.

Bellenger, M. C. (2017). *Prendre au « sérieux » les loisirs de prédation: Chasse, pêche, cueillette et naturalisme dans l'estuaire de la Seine.* PhD Thesis, CETAPS, Université de Rouen Normandie.

Bendle, L. J., & Pooley, A. W. (2016). Higher skilled working tourists and their leisure lifestyles: A qualitative study of guest language instructors in South Korea. *Leisure Studies, 35*, 406–420. https://doi.org/10.1080/02614367.2014.967712

Chen, H., Xi, L., & Zhao, J. (2018). Work values, satisfaction and self-efficacy of college student voluntourists in southern China. *International Journal of Marketing Studies, 10*(4), 86–93. https://doi.org/10.5539/ijms.v10n4p86

Court, K. (2020). Knitting two together (k2tog), "if you meet another knitter you always have a friend". *Textile, 18*(3), 278–291. https://doi.org/10.1080/14759756.2019.1690838

Davidson, L., & Stebbins, R. A. (2011). *Serious leisure and nature: Sustainable consumption in the outdoors.* Palgrave Macmillan.

Fine, G. A. (1998). *Morel tales: The culture of mushrooming.* Harvard University Press.

Frew, E. A. (2006). Comedy festival attendance: Serious, project-based or casual leisure? In S. Elkington, I. Jones, & L. Lawrence (Eds.), *Serious leisure: Extensions and applications* (pp. 105–122). LSA Publications, University of Brighton.

Gravelle, F., & Larocque, L. (2005). Volunteerism and serious leisure: The case of the francophone games. *World Leisure Journal, 47*(1), 45–51.

Hershkovitz, A., & Hardof-Jaffe, S. (2017). Genealogy as a lifelong endeavor. *Leisure/Loisir, 41*(4), 535–560.

Palso, N. T. (2008). *Serious road-tripping: A study of serious and project-based leisure in self-drive recreationists in Alaska.* Doctoral thesis, Department of Recreation, Parks, and Tourism Management, Pennsylvania State University (USA).

Presser, L., & Taylor, W. V. (2011). An autoethnography of hunting. *Crime, Law and Social Change, 55*(5), 483–494.

Rossetti, G., & Quinn, B. (2023). The value of the serious leisure perspective in understanding cultural capital embodiment in festival settings. *The Sociological Review, 71*(3), 526–543. https://doi.org/10.1177/00380261221108589

Roued, H., Castenbrandt, H., & Revuelta-Eugercio, B. A. (2023). Search, save and share: Family historians' engagement practices with digital platforms. *Archival Science, 23*, 187–120. https://doi.org/10.1007/s10502-022-09404-413

Segal, N. (2022). Ukrainians turn to diaries for solace, and to share life in wartime. *New York Times*, 4 November, online edition.

Stalp, M. B. (2007). *Quilting: The fabric of everyday life*. Berg.

Stebbins, R. A. (1994). The liberal arts hobbies: A neglected subtype of serious leisure. *Loisir et Société/Society and Leisure, 16*, 173–186.

Stebbins, R. A. (2014). *Careers in serious leisure: From dabbler to devotee in search of fulfillment*. Palgrave Macmillan.

Strong, W. (2022). Family of 4 makes 1500 km journey through N.W.T. backcountry. *CBC News* (22 September), https://www.cbc.ca/news/canada/north/nwt-backcountry-travel-with-youngsters-1.5292099.

Twynam, G. D., Farrell, J. M., & Johnston, M. E. (2002/2003). Leisure and volunteer motivation at a special sporting event. *Leisure/Loisir, 27*, 363–377.

Undlien, R. (2019). Lasting social value or a one-off? People with intellectual disabilities' experiences with volunteering for the Youth Olympic Games. *Journal of Sport for Development, 7*(13), 33–45.

Warner, A., Callaghan, E., & de Vreede, C. (2014). Promoting sustainable food and food citizenship through an adult education leisure experience. *Leisure/Loisir, 37*, 337–360. https://doi.org/10.1080/02614367.2014.993334

Wensing, E. (2020). *Crafty commemoration: Vernacular responses to the Centenary of World War One*. PhD thesis, Australian National University, Canberra.

Wichmann, A. (2017). Participating in the World Gymnaestrada: An expression and experience of community. *Leisure Studies, 36*, 21–38. https://doi.org/10.1080/02614367.2015.1052836

Chapter 3
Project-Based Leisure as Obligation

Abstract This chapter opens with a discussion of agreeable versus disagreeable obligation. The agreeable project-based variety is occasionally found in making something, as in a swing hung from a tree for a child's pleasure or a special meal with which to celebrate a birthday. Volunteering on a project basis can be moderately agreeable. Some fine artists get drawn into one-off projects that fall outside their routine involvements. Theatrical skills may be especially relevant here, as in being invited to emcee a talent show or variety-arts show or serve as a chairperson for a set of scholarly conference papers.

Keywords Agreeable vs. disagreeable obligation · Making things · Volunteering · Fine arts one-off projects · Leisure and volunteering · Personal projects

This chapter opens with a discussion of agreeable versus disagreeable obligation. The agreeable project-based variety is occasionally found in making something, as in a swing hung from a tree for a child's pleasure or a special meal with which to celebrate a birthday. Volunteering on a project basis can be moderately agreeable, for example, participating in a roadside clean-up campaign and chaperoning a school dance. Some fine artists get drawn into one-off projects that fall outside their routine involvements. Theatrical skills may be especially relevant here, as in being invited to emcee a talent show or variety-arts show or serve as a chairperson for a set of scholarly conference papers. Moreover, the word "obligation" has a puzzling ring to it when bandied about in leisure circles. For one, it generates a sense of having to do something or think in some way; someone is obliged to do such and such, which that person may not want to do. This is obligation in its negative sense. In contrast with this meaning is the sense that obligation is part of doing something one likes to do, as in showing up to play a game of basketball with one's team, acting a part in a play, and filling an exciting volunteer role (Stebbins, 2001). Here obligation is positive, it is an agreeable responsibility.

Two Types of Obligation

The word "obligation" has a puzzling ring to it when bandied about in leisure circles. For one, it generates a sense of having to do something or think in some way; someone is obliged to do such and such, which that person may not want to do. This is obligation in its negative sense. In contrast with this meaning is the sense that obligation is part of doing something one likes to do, as in showing up to play a game of basketball with one's team, acting a part in a play, and filling an exciting volunteer role (Stebbins, 2001). Here obligation is positive, it is an agreeable responsibility.

Some of the earliest theoretic stirrings in this area came from Philip Bosserman and Richard Gagan (1972, p. 115) and from David Horton Smith (1975, p. 148) all of whom argued that, at the level of the individual, all leisure activity is voluntary action. More precise statements were made about the same time and somewhat later by Max Kaplan (1975, p. 394) and John Neulinger (1981, p. 19), two leisure studies specialists, who observed in passing how leisure can serve either oneself or other people, if not both (see also Smith, 1981; Kelly, 1990) . It is presumed that they had volunteerism in mind, even though some amateur and hobbyist activities also have this dual function (e.g., community music and theater and sports like curling and ice and powerboat racing). From the side of voluntary action research, Kenneth Boulding (1973, p. 31) theorized that voluntary service borders on leisure, frequently even overlapping it. Alex Dickson (1974, p. xiii) observed that leisure is seen in commonsense as part of voluntary action and does in fact "carry this spare-time connotation."

As mentioned earlier, we also daydream or ponder more seriously at times and more long-term about how to escape some of these unpleasant aspects of life. For example, Homo obligatus hopes that by next year his divorce proceedings will at last be settled or by that time he will have enough money to buy a better car to replace the present one that keeps breaking down. These obligations are met in non-work time, but thoughts about them may emerge in the other.

The World of Leisure Projects

Before taking up our discussion of PBL and obligation, we need first to gain a sense of the larger world of its diverse on-off projects. In all these projects people generally use the talents and knowledge they have at hand, even though for some projects they may seek certain instructions beforehand, including reading a manual or taking a short course. And some projects resembling hobbyist activity participation may require a modicum of preliminary conditioning. Always, the goal is to undertake successfully the one-off project and nothing more, and sometimes a small amount of background preparation is necessary for this. It is possible that a survey would show that most project-based leisure is hobbyist in character and the next most common, a kind of volunteering. First, the following hobbyist-like projects have so far been identified:[1]

- Making and tinkering:

    - Interlacing, interlocking, and knot-making from kits
    - Other kit assembly projects (e.g., stereo tuner, craft store projects, quilts, beer)
    - Do-it-yourself projects done primarily for fulfillment, some of which may even be undertaken with minimal skill and knowledge (e.g., build a rock wall or a fence, finish a room in the basement, plant a special garden). This could turn into an irregular series of such projects, spread over many years, possibly even transforming the participant into a hobbyist.

- Liberal arts:

    - Genealogy (not as ongoing hobby)
    - Tourism: special trip, not as part of an extensive personal tour program, to visit different parts of a region, a continent, or much of the world

- Activity participation: long back-packing trip, canoe trip; one-off mountain ascent (e.g., Fuji, Rainier, Kilimanjaro)

One-off volunteering projects are also common, though possibly somewhat less so than hobbyist-like projects. And less common than either are the amateur-like projects, which seem to concentrate in the sphere of theater.

- Volunteering

    - Volunteer at a convention or conference, whether local, national, or international in scope.
    - Volunteer at a sporting competition, whether local, national, or international in scope.
    - Volunteer at an arts festival or special exhibition mounted in a museum or heritage site.
    - Volunteer to help restore human life or wildlife after a natural or human-made disaster caused by, for instance, a hurricane, earthquake, oil spill, or industrial accident.

- Arts projects:

    - Entertainment theatre: produce a skit or one-off community pageant; prepare a home film, video or set of photos.
    - Public speaking: prepare a talk for a reunion, an after-dinner speech, an oral position statement on an issue to be discussed at a community meeting.
    - Memoirs: therapeutic audio, visual and written productions by the elderly; life histories and autobiographies (all ages); accounts of personal events (all ages) (Stebbins, 2011).

---

[1] The remainder this section is taken with added updates from Stebbins (2005, pp. 5–6)

Making Something

A couple of examples appeared in the introduction to this chapter, namely, making and hanging a swing and preparing a special meal for a special occasion. Both rewards and costs were mentioned by my interviewees during research into their serious pursuits. More particularly, they saw their leisure as a mix of rewards offsetting costs as experienced in the central activity. Moreover, every serious pursuit contains its own combination of these costs, which each participant must confront in some way. In other words, costs are motivators—we are motivated to avoid them (Stebbins, 2020, p. 30).

Exterior Home Projects

These fall into two broad categories: outside the home (its exterior and adjacent property) and inside the home be it either a house or an apartment. Garden projects—for example, stone/brick formations; planters, trellises; layouts of plants, shrubs, and pathways—are common among homeowners with sufficient space for growing things. The hobby in question here is gardening consisting, in the main, of regular planting, weeding, watering, fertilizing, trimming (shrubs, small trees), warding off pests, gathering flowers, and harvesting vegetables, berries or tree fruits (e.g., Cheng et al., 2017; Scott et al., 2020).

These activities, which are repeated off and on during the growing season, fall within the core activity of gardening. Outside it the hobbyist may also undertake certain agreeable projects, such as the ones just mentioned. They either augment or enhance this core activity in diverse ways, thereby giving them positive appeal rather than seeing them as a nonwork obligation. Thus, a flagstone pathway throughout the garden area augments access to it, whereas planters and trellises enhance the beauty of the flora contained within.

Backyard bird houses and feeders augment the opportunity to observe some of the local avian wildlife. Annually decorating the front yard with lights, structures, and personages related to Halloween and Christmas exemplifies occasional PBL. Certain national holidays and similar personal celebrations inspire some individuals to mount annually occasional agreeable projects consisting of an ensemble of inventive element. Personal announcements may get expressed as PBL in signs aimed at passers-by, as seen in special birthdays (e.g., Lordy Lordy John is Forty), political preferences (e.g., We Support the X Amendment), among others. In this vein see Zedd (2022) for a multitude of additional examples.

Inner-Home Projects

Depending on the outlook of the participant, hanging a new set of curtains or blinds or repainting in one or more rooms can be PBL. The same may be said for DIY-level tiling of, say, bathroom or kitchen floors. What might transform a possible tiling leisure project into a nonwork obligation or a search for professional help are thoughts about the difficulty of removing the old flooring. Such doubts are sown in even greater quantity when contemplating developing the basement of one's home. A multitude of trade-related activities must be considered, among them electricity, carpentry, dry-wall construction, ceiling and lighting, and flooring. Thus basement development may, upon study from the SLP, turnout to be more often nonwork obligation than PBL.

Constructing a genealogy is in substantial part a home-based activity and commonly, it appears, a one-off undertaking. In other words, hobbyist genealogists are interested in the history of their own families, which tackled on a part-time basis is usually a multi-year affair (Horne, 2008; Darby & Clough, 2013; Hershkovitz & Hardof-Jaffe, 2017). Ideally, these hobbyists will find the time and the money to visit distant (often foreign) communities in search of critical information on relevant dates (e.g., birth, death, marriage), status (e.g., occupational, community, marital), levels of education, and the like.

For those who are mechanically inclined, they might consider a DIY tech project. Marguerite Preston (2023) describes the "Raspberry Pi":

> a pocket-sized Linux computer that can be programmed and adapted with accessories to do all kinds of things. With a little patience and know-how, you can make it operate as a VPN, turn it into a camera, or make a DIY voice assistant. We also have a guide to turning the Raspberry Pi into a retro-gaming console, which you can do in about half an hour with a few accessories.

Preston recommends that most people acquire the "CanaKit Raspberry Pi 4 Starter Kit," that is unless they plan to build a game console. In this case they should stick with the Raspberry Pi 3. That kit includes the fastest Raspberry Pi model that her team tested, as well as almost everything else one needs to get started. The participant does have to supply a keyboard, mouse, and screen. Other project ideas and tutorials can be found on the websites of Make Magazine Adafruit Industries, Instructables.com, and The MagPi. Other outside-the-home projects involve in Making something include glassblowing (O'Connor, 2007), dowsing, and kite-making and flying.

Volunteer Projects

Volunteering on a project basis can be most agreeable, for example, one-time participation in a roadside clean-up campaign and chaperoning a school dance. Some fine artists get drawn into one-off projects that fall outside their routine involvements. Theatrical skills may be especially relevant on such occasions, as in being invited to emcee a show displaying talent or a range of the variety-arts or serving as chairperson of a session of scholarly talks.

Mentoring has been conceptualized as a distinctive kind of serious leisure volunteering (Stebbins, 2006), since it leads to a unique career in a leisure activity. That is, mentoring stands apart from tutoring, coaching, and the like, in part, because the former lasts significantly longer both as a role and as a foundation for a deep interpersonal relationship. As in all volunteering—this holds, too, for tutoring, teaching, and coaching—there is also a target of benefits, referred to here as the protégé. But only mentoring is substantially motivated by a focused altruism, a strongly held attitude that disposes the mentor to help another because of concern for that person's welfare or satisfaction, if not both.

Though altruism is a quintessential feature of volunteering, research nevertheless makes clear that, generally, volunteering is also characterised by a self-serving, self-interested component. So this altruism is, in effect, "relative altruism," with "pure, other-serving altruism" being extremely rare (Smith, 2000). It is the self-interested facet of altruism that brings us to the leisure qualities of both it and mentoring. All leisure, the serious form most certainly included, is self-interested activity.

Defining the Work-Leisure Axis of Volunteering[2]

Notwithstanding these misconceptions it is possible to marry the economic and leisure understandings of volunteering. Let us start by observing that the first is, in part, descriptive; it portrays volunteering as, at bottom, intentionally-productive unpaid work. But one problem with this blanket qualification is that by no means all such work is voluntary, as the domain of non-work obligation so clearly shows (activities in this domain are by definition disagreeable, the agreeable ones being essentially leisure, Stebbins, 2009, Chap. 1). Moreover, some other kinds of unpaid work hardly resemble paid work, since they are essentially leisure. Is it not true, then, that a principal attraction of this economic conception is its capacity to steer attention to an important sphere of life beyond employment, beyond livelihood?

Note further that I have described the unpaid work in question as *intentionally-productive*. In volunteering volunteers intend to generate something of value for both self and other (non-family) individuals, or their group, or their community, if not a combination of these three. The various examples offered in the preceding sections attest both this intention and, in these instances, its productive outcome. Moreover, the concept of intentionally-productive unpaid work occupies some common ground with the SLP. The latter, particularly in its serious leisure and project-based forms, includes a set of ten personal and social rewards that participants may realize through participation in the activities the forms subsume (Stebbins,

---

[2]The early paragraphs of this section were paraphrased from Stebbins (2013, p. 341).

1996, 2007, pp. 13–17). In other words, unpaid volunteer work, when productive, leads to these benefits for self (i.e., intrinsic "psychic benefits" and possibly extrinsic instrumental payoffs) as well as for other individuals, groups, or the community as a whole.

It is this second quality of the idea of unpaid work *as* intended productivity that carries it beyond description into explanation. Such work is supposed to produce results, thereby showing the utility of volunteering. Furthermore, now on the explanatory level, the definitional ball gets passed to leisure.

Leisure's Contribution

A definition of leisure that goes well with the present discussion is the one presented in Chap. 1: leisure is un-coerced, contextually framed activity engaged in during free time, which people want to do and, using their abilities and resources, actually do in either a satisfying or a fulfilling way (or both). This definition applies to all three SLP forms and the types of volunteering they subsume. Let us dissect it.

First, leisure is un-coerced, felt to be such by the participant pursing it. So it is with unpaid work as well, to the extent the "worker" feels the same way. Nonetheless, if people are driven by strong moral imperatives to work without remuneration, Freeman's (1997, S141) observations suggest that they are coerced and therefore not engaged in leisure:

> Many people volunteer in response to a request to do so. Their behaviour is not 'volunteering' in the dictionary sense of offering one's services freely but rather its opposite: exceeding to requests. From this perspective, voluntary and other charitable activity that people do largely when asked are 'conscience goods': public goods to which people give time or money because they recognize the moral case for doing so and to which they feel social pressure to undertake when asked, but whose provision they would just as soon let someone else do.

They are faced instead with a non-work obligation. But can people be morally driven to do something they also like to do, for instance, the fathers in the following common division of domestic labor in the West?

> Childcare is unpaid work, during which women devote most of their time with children to the physical care of the latter, especially cooking and cleaning up after meals. By contrast, men performing childcare do this by teaching, reading, and playing with their young ones. Viewed from the SLP, the women are caught in a daily grind of *non-work obligation* (this assumes they dislike routine family cooking and dishwashing), whereas their husbands or partners enjoy serious leisure *hobbyist* time with their children. In fact, because the target of benefits is one's family, such activities according to some definitions of the term might not even be considered volunteering. (Stebbins, 2013, pp. 340–341)

Is this not, for the father, effectively leisure activity? I believe the logic of our argument here forces us to answer this question affirmatively. In other words, *agreeable* non-work obligation is essentially leisure (for more examples see

Stebbins, 2009, pp. 53–54). Note, however, that the father's leisure here is not volunteering, for it is found within his family.

Second, leisure is contextually framed; placed in the social, cultural, historical circumstances of the activity being pursued. Is volunteering done for an organization, small group, friend, social movement, the wider community? Is it formal or is it informal, as in helping someone? When joined with relevant cultural and historical conditions, we have added another major explanatory slant to our definition of work-leisure in volunteering. The free time in which all this unfolds refers to those hours not spent performing either paid work or unpleasant, non-work obligations. This has been identified as the temporal context of leisure, and it includes volunteering as unpaid work (Stebbins, 2012).

Third, people want to enjoy their leisure activities. Yet, it is difficult to discern this motivational theme in the concept of unpaid work, which as it stands, forces the question of why "work" for no pay at all? The answer, in general, is that people want to do such activity. In particular they want to realize the aforementioned personal and social rewards that the activity offers them, accomplishing this by using their abilities and resources to pursue either satisfying casual leisure or fulfilling serious or project-based leisure.

Personal Projects

Earning a bachelor's degree or, for some, even a (non-thesis) master's is a leisure project rather than a stepping-stone on the long route (for some people) to a decent livelihood. For the first the degree represents a recognized level of mastery of the program's course material, since the project is one of self-development rather than a means to finding an occupational career. In other words, earning a bachelor's degree to further oneself is a kind of liberal arts undertaking, and indeed, may be a special part of a liberal arts hobby in, say, literature or history. In Britain Jonathan Hallow has made getting a doctorate in literature a main PBL pursuit in his early retirement (Nelson, 2023).

In another area of life consider the project of landing a marital partner, including strategies for making and maintaining contact with the object of affection, finding common ground in matters of mutual interest, learning about the background of family and friends, and the like. To this sub-type we may add such time-limited undertakings as surprise birthday parties, elaborate preparations for a major holiday, and volunteering for sports events.

Furthermore, since social worlds are enduring phenomena, they cannot by definition be found in project-based leisure, commonly an evanescent interest (Stebbins, 2018, p. 8). This may seem arbitrary, for strangers supplying material and services may be necessary in making something (e.g., a rock garden, a playroom in the basement, a macramé decoration) and tourists may become involved as appreciators of the finished project. But, critically, there are few if any members (regular or insider) to constitute a social world centered on a project, given that projects are usually one-person undertakings or more rarely two or three other people who just for that project help build a garage, prepare a wedding reception, put on a skit, or take a canoe trip.

This said a rudimentary social world does begin to develop around certain complex PBL projects (Stebbins, 2018). Each in its own way brings together as participants friends, neighbors, or relatives (e.g., drawn together by a genealogical project or elaborate Christmas or Halloween displays), or pull the individual enthusiast into an organizational milieu (e.g., through one-time volunteering for a sports event, major convention, or arts festival).

Worth exploring in future research, given that some obligations can be pleasant and attractive, is the nature and extent of leisure-like projects carried out within the context of paid employment. Furthermore, this discussion jibes with the additional criterion that the project, to qualify as project-based leisure, must be seen by the project creator as fundamentally uncoerced, fulfilling activity. Finally, note that project-based leisure cannot, by definition, refer to projects carried out as part of a person's serious leisure, such as mounting a star night as an amateur astronomer or a model train display as a collector.

The closest conceptual relative to project-based leisure turns up in personality psychology under the heading of 'personal projects'. Brian Little, author of this idea, defines them as:

> ... extended sets of personally relevant action, which range from the trivial pursuits of a typical Tuesday (e.g., 'cleaning up my room') to the magnificent obsessions of a lifetime (e.g., 'liberate my people'). They may be self-initiated or thrust upon us. They may be solitary concerns or shared commitments. They may be isolated and peripheral aspects of our lives or may cut to our very core. Personal projects may sustain us through perplexity or serve as vehicles for our own obliteration. In short, personal projects are natural units of analysis for a personality psychology that chooses to deal with the serious business of how people muddle through complex lives. (Little, 1989, p. 15).

Our concern here with leisure projects is clearly only one, albeit important, part of the vast domain of personal projects studied by Little and colleagues. Since their research does not distinguish personal projects according to whether they are leisure or something else, what we can learn through future explorations of project-based leisure should contribute substantially to this branch of psychology, as it also should to the field of leisure studies.

Payette and Chrétien (2023) studied "equicoaching" workshops as PBL/personal projects for riders and trainors:

> The equicoaching workshops awarded our collaborators with opportunities to both interact with horses, on the ground, and to discuss work–life boundary management issues, past and present. Workshops included: education on general horse behavior and proper handling maneuvers, grooming sessions, experiencing "being part of the herd," and activities around various modules. Concerning these modules, and as will be explained below, the general idea is to get horses to interact with various materials and obstacles (smell them, step on them, or walk through them) (p. 6).

Conclusions

Clearly, not all projects in life are pursued as leisure. One prominent category in this set is made up of those that are medical. Replacement of, say, a hip or a knee, removal of a cataract, or augmentation of both breasts number among these projects, which in the language of the SLP are usually of the non-work variety (for the patient). They are not PBL. The principal actors here are the medical team and the patient, wherein the latter must follow such instructions as swallow certain medications, wear certain corrective clothing or devices, and exercise properly the bodily part involved.

Other non-work obligations can be as disagreeable and enduring as the medical kind. Getting a divorce, buying a house, or paying off a large student loan are examples. Furthermore, meeting them cuts into temporal and financial resources that might otherwise be devoted leisure interests. Some of those interests may be one-off contributions to the community.

References

Bosserman, P., & Gagan, R. (1972). Leisure and voluntary action. In D. H. Smith (Ed.), *Voluntary action research: 1972* (pp. 109–126). D.C. Heath.

Boulding, K. (1973). *The economy of love and fear*. Wadsworth.

Cheng, E., Stebbins, R., & Packer, J. (2017). Serious leisure among older gardeners in Australia. *Leisure Studies, 36*(4), 505–518.

Darby, P., & Clough, P. (2013). Investigating the information-seeking behaviour of genealogists and family historians. *Journal of Information Science, 39*(1), 73–84.

Dickson, A. (1974). Foreword. In D. H. Smith (Ed.), *Voluntary action research: 1974* (pp. xiii–xx). D.C. Heath.

Freeman, R. B. (1997). Working for nothing: The supply of volunteer labor. *Journal of Labor Economics, 15*, S140–S166.

Hershkovitz, A., & Hardof-Jaffe, S. (2017). Genealogy as a lifelong endeavor. *Leisure/Loisir, 41*(4), 535–560.

Horne, A. J. (2008). *Genealogy mania*. VDM Verlag Dr. Müller.

Kaplan, M. (1975). *Leisure: Theory and policy*. Wiley.

Kelly, J. R. (1990). *Leisure* (2nd ed.). Prentice Hall.

Little, B. R. (1989). Personal projects analysis: Trivial pursuits, magnificent obsessions, and the search for coherence. In D. M. Buss & N. Cantor (Eds.), *Personality psychology*. Springer. https://doi.org/10.1007/978-1-4684-0634-4_2

Nelson, E. (2023). Britain wants its early retirees back, but their days are 'never boring.' *New Work Times*, Thursday 14 March.

Neulinger, J. (1981). *The psychology of leisure* (2nd ed.). Charles C. Thomas.

O'Connor, E. (2007). Embodied knowledge in glassblowing: The experience of meaning and the struggle towards proficiency. *The Sociological Review, 55*(1-supp), 126–141. https://doi.org/10.1111/j.1467-954X.2007.00697.x

Payette, B., & Chrétien, L. (2023). How meeting with the horse may contribute to a balanced life: Co-constructing a project-based leisure. *Loisir et Société/Society and Leisure*. https://doi.org/10.1080/07053436.2023.2216586

Preston, M. (2023). 5 simple ways to start a new hobby while staying home. *New York Times*, 8 February, online edition.

Scott, T. L., Masser, B. M., & Pachana, N. A. (2020). Positive aging benefits of home and community gardening activities: Older adults report enhanced self-esteem, productive endeavours, social engagement and exercise. *Sage Open Medicine, 8*, 1–13. https://doi.org/10.1177/2050312120901732

Smith, D. H. (1975). Voluntary action and voluntary groups. In A. Inkeles, J. Coleman, & N. Smelser (Eds.), *Annual review of sociology* (Vol. 1, pp. 247–270). Annual Reviews Inc.

Smith, D. H. (1981). Altruism, volunteers, and volunteerism. *Journal of Voluntary Action Research, 10*, 21–36.

Smith, D. H. (2000). *Grassroots associations*. Sage.

Stebbins, R. A. (1996). Volunteering: A serious leisure perspective. *Nonprofit and Voluntary Sector Quarterly, 25*, 211–224.

Stebbins, R. A. (2001). Volunteering – mainstream and marginal: Preserving the leisure experience. In M. Graham & M. Foley (Eds.), *Volunteering in leisure: Marginal or inclusive?* (Vol. 75, pp. 1–10). Leisure Studies Association.

Stebbins, R. A. (2005). Project-based leisure: Theoretical neglect of a common use of free time. *Leisure Studies, 24*, 1–11.

Stebbins, R. A. (2006). Mentoring as a leisure activity: On the informal world of small-scale altruism. *World Leisure Journal, 48*(4), 3–10.

Stebbins, R. A. (2007). *Serious leisure: A perspective for our time*. New Brunswick, NJ/New York: Transaction/Routledge, 2017, paperback edition with new Preface.

Stebbins, R. A. (2009). *Personal decisions in the public square: Beyond problem solving into a positive sociology* (p. 2017). Transaction/Routledge.

Stebbins, R. A. (2011). Paid to volunteer: The monetary consideration in defining volunteering. *e-Volunteerism: A Journal to Inform and Challenge Leaders of Volunteers, 11*(2) online publication.

Stebbins, R. A. (2012). *The idea of leisure: First principles* (p. 2017). Transaction/Routledge.

Stebbins, R. A. (2013). Unpaid work of love: Defining the work-leisure axis of volunteering. *Leisure Studies, 32*(3), 339–345.

Stebbins, R. A. (2018). *Social worlds and the leisure experience*. Emerald Group.

Stebbins, R. (2020). *The serious leisure perspective: A synthesis*. Palgrave Macmillan.

Zedd, C. (2022). *Get off my lawn: Check out the most hilarious signs neighbors hung in their yards (23 November)*. https://theprimarymarket.com/signs-neighbors-hung-in-their-b0?utm_source=mediago-b0&utm_medium=&utm_campaign=b0-ca-d-tp

Chapter 4
One-Off Contributions to the Community

Abstract One-off contributions to the community are PBL when its members volunteer in a local disaster recovery or neighborhood clean-up, decoration, or gardening project. Neighbors may meet on one or more occasions to craft a solution to a local problem, such as road repair or excessive traffic. Hobbyist project volunteering is evident in coin and model railroad displays. And voluntourism in a developing country is often undertaken for a period of a few days to three to six months. Typically, these volunteers work with a charity in a PBL activity building (houses, providing health care, or serving in schools. One-off volunteering, pure or mixed with amateur or hobbyist interests, is clearly a main way of engaging in community-related PBL. Still, the community served through PBL can also be conceived of in much narrower terms, as in knitting sweaters and mittens for grandchildren and baking cookies and cakes for the extended family.

Keywords episodic volunteering · local emergencies · role of volunteer in a disaster · voluntourism · neighborhood cleanup and decoration · local problems · hobbyist-like PBL

One-off contributions to the community are PBL when its members volunteer in a local disaster recovery or neighborhood clean-up, decoration, or gardening project. Neighbors may meet on one or more occasions to craft a solution to a local problem, such as road repair or excessive traffic. Hobbyist project volunteering is evident in coin and model railroad displays. And voluntourism in a developing country is often undertaken for a period of few days to 3–6 months. Typically, these volunteers work with a charity in a PBL activity building (houses, providing health care, or serving in schools. We examine all four of these in this chapter.

Episodic Volunteering

An episodic volunteer is committed to working only for a short time, usually several days or weeks, rather than committed to working for, say, 6 months to a year. Episodic volunteers may do the same short-term volunteer work on a regular annual basis or may do so only once, basically as PBL (Macduff, 1991). This conception contrasts with that of the continuous service volunteer.

Holmes (2014) has noted the prominent role of episodic volunteers in tourism some of whom engage in PBL. She found that the retired episodic volunteers she interviewed did not have the same complex commitments as employed respondents but still did not want to be tied down to a regular volunteer role. In other words, for them diverse additional leisure activities also beckon and time must be set aside for them as well.

Local Emergencies

It is the "spontaneous volunteer"—a type of episodic voluntourism—who responds to local emergencies and is defined by Smith et al. (2006, p. 218) as:

> one who helps . . . out at a disaster site (natural or human-made) so-called because motivation to do so emerges at the moment of learning about the disaster. Such a person, who may have come from afar, may not possess the skills needed at the disaster site, and may not be wanted there, is likely to abandon this role after having served there.

Such volunteers, people usually motivated by the emotional impact of the disaster itself, are typically unaffiliated with organizations devoted to disaster relief (e.g., the Red Cross).

The disaster in question—a hurricane, tornado, earthquake, oil spill, forest fire, flood, industrial accident—is local in the sense that the would-be volunteer can reach the site reasonably easily as well as strongly identify with it. And the volunteer in question is the volitional type defined in Chap. 1, who by the way, is most likely to be pursuing a casual leisure activity rather than one that is serious (i.e., career leisure volunteering).

Role of the Volunteer in a Disaster

Volunteer Canada (https://volunteer.ca/index.php?MenuItemID=390) states that

> no two-disaster management or recovery situations are the same. Factors include the amount of forewarning issued to the community, the preparedness of local citizens (e.g., stores of water, food), emergency infrastructure (e.g., hurricane shelters), and the capacity and coordination of local emergency response agencies (e.g. police, fire, shelters, charities/ NGOs, government departments). Also, the kind of response required changes as the

situation progresses. For example, preparation for a hurricane, when the hurricane touches down, the period of immediate emergency support to persons in danger, support to persons in shelters following a hurricane who have lost homes, water contamination and power structure damage all require different skills and changing leadership amongst emergency response agencies. The well-meaning involvement of agencies or individuals that have not been a part of the coordinated response effort at each of these stages can impede, rather than support, recovery.

When should you go into a disaster to help?

Those wishing to volunteer in an emergency situation must look to the (often evolving) requests of the coordinating agencies for what support they need and when. Usually, those agencies want pre-trained individuals. For example, volunteers wishing to help in Florida immediately after a hurricane are usually required to have shelter volunteer training and a background check, according to Volunteer Florida. When calling for volunteer support in a disaster, the Canadian Red Cross often requires volunteers to have received their emergency management volunteer training. Coordinating agencies often issue urgent requests for volunteers trained in emergency response (e.g. fire, police) and medical personnel (e.g. nurse and doctors) to increase local capacity. In sum, unless you have received the training requested by coordinating agencies, don't go. You might not only be in the way, you may be putting your own safety at risk, adding to the emergency.

Similar requirements, organizations, and needs for spontaneous volunteers exist in most modern industrial societies.

Other Voluntourism

Habitat for Humanity International is a well-known example of this kind of volunteering often, it appears, to be of the PBL variety. That is, here participants commit themselves to 6–12 months of voluntary construction of housing in a developing country where such is in short supply. Even more demanding are the requirements of the Peace Corps in the United States, which asks for 3 months of training followed by at least 2 years of service in the developing world. Since most of the volunteers in this area are young adults, they are unlikely to sign up for another session of service here. For them their single session is PBL is to be followed by gainful employment back in their home country.

Shannon Woodward (2007) recounts the experiences of eight Canadians who spent 6 months in several countries in Africa and Asia providing clean water. To accomplish this, they built biosand water filters. The participants were on a "Water for Life" internship sponsored by Samaritan's Purse.

WorldTeach is a non-profit NGO that provides opportunities for volunteers to make meaningful contributions to international education by living and teaching in non-Western countries (www.worldteach.org). Volunteers pay a fee that covers return airfare and cost of living. Teaching opportunities are often offered on a 2-months basis over the summer. Semester and year-long assignments are also available.

Wearing (2004) examines voluntourism more generally. Besides community development in non-Western societies, it includes projects in science and medicine carried out there. Under the rubric of science we find volunteering centered on issues in the physical environment and public health. Moreover, these volunteers often help out on matters of personal health (e.g., sanitation, eye care) and education (e.g., language acquisition, reading skills). Americorps VISTA, for example, offers summer volunteer programs, though only in the USA. Such PBL is of 3–4 months duration (between May and September) when most university students are not taking classes.

Neighborhood Cleanup and Decoration

This section bears on a one-off activity that may seem relatively inconsequential, namely, gathering together a group to clean up a neighborhood for a day or two (from Community Tool Box, https://ctb.ku.edu/en/table-of-contents/implement/physical-social-environment/neighborhood-cleanup-programs/main). Note, however, that a neighborhood cleanup can have a strong positive impact, particularly on low-income neighborhoods whose residents seldom see anything better in their future. Both engaging in the cleanup and seeing its results can change a neighborhood's culture and self-image, leading residents to view themselves in a different light.

A neighborhood cleanup as described here may be led by the community, by an organized neighborhood association or council, by a grass roots neighborhood group, or by one or more concerned individuals. They undertake three kinds of neighborhood cleanups, any or all of which can be carried out in a single one-off event:

- Public space cleanup. Neighborhood volunteers, usually with simple equipment—brooms, shovels, gloves, trash bags—spend some or all of a day cleaning up part or all of a neighborhood.
- Household cleanup. On a designated day or week, neighborhood volunteers or the municipality will (usually at no cost to the household) pick up items too large for regular waste disposal or otherwise difficult to get rid of. Residents simply leave the items waiting to be picked up at the edge of the road at an appointed date and time.
- Community-assisted cleanup. If one of the spots most in need of a cleanup is on private property—a vacant lot in which the owner or others have dumped a large amount of trash and bulky waste, for example—or if there are items, such as abandoned or junked cars, that a neighborhood group simply can't remove, the neighborhood may need help from the larger community. The municipality may be able to provide permits, equipment, and other aids to address the problem.

Turning to decoration, that related to the Christmas, Halloween, and Easter seasons featured as a part of a neighborhood, its entry, or its parkland is sometimes a community project rather than a personal project as described in Chap. 3. Such requires a plan, organization of help, and commitment on the part of the helpers. The latter includes also being available to disassemble the project when the special season has passed. To the extent that participants become involved in this kind of PBL, they may choose to so as a one-shot affair or as a hobby pursued over the years.

Local Problems

Depending on where the participant lives local problems can seem innumerable. Road repair and excessive traffic have already been mentioned, while others may include neighborhood crime, snow clearance, barking dogs, unsightly properties, and obnoxious noise (often loud music, late-night parties). The first two in this list along with snow clearance, barking dogs, and unsightly property are typically matters to be considered by the municipal council, thus requiring one or more indignant members of the neighborhood to bring their problem to its attention. This initial contact may not be sufficient, however, since the problem continues. Next steps could include getting more property holders in the neighborhood to contact the council or to write their councilor.

Winnipegger, Debbie Collins, found herself in this situation living two doors down from two dogs in the Crestview area.

"[The owners] would leave them outside all day long and the poor things would bark and bark and bark and bark," Collins said. "I wasn't mad at the dogs—I was more mad at the owners."

Collins said she filed three complaints with the city's Animal Services after the barking went on for months.

The dogs yapped and cried as Collins watched her alarm clock tick closer to her morning alarm.

She had enough and marched to the house in her housecoat.

"I said, 'you need to let your dogs in, they have been barking for eight hours,'" Collins explained. "And I turned around to leave and the woman said, 'oh, they're outside?'"

A frustrated Collins told her neighbour she would be back with Animal Services. She doesn't know if city officials dealt with her complaints, but Collins said after the conversation with the woman, the dogs stopped barking. (Carty, 2017)

Eventually the neighbours moved away.

Other local problems can be more difficult to solve, which turns them into a prolonged PBL. Break and entry, auto theft, gun violence, and physical assault are illegal and demand thus legal remedy. New bylaws may be needed, legal counsel may be necessary, and petitions and opinion polls can show the level of community support for solutions to them. Setting these complex processes in motion takes time and takes even more time for them to run their course. As part of a leisure project, each directly involves the participant though only sporadically from start to finish. Moreover, each qualifies as volunteering of the PBL kind.

Hobbyist-Like PBL

Hobbyist-like project-based volunteering is evident in, among others, coin and model railroad displays. Coin shows abound often sponsored by local numismatic societies and sometimes also featuring stamps and possibly medals. Here enthusiasts can buy, sell, or trade sought-after coins (and paper currency, medals), stamps, and so on as they strive to enrich their collections. This is what these hobbyists do as hobbyists (Case, 2009). As a hobbyist-like PBL, a one-off activity, could be displaying one's own collection at an annual convention or show (usually local), or doing this so infrequently that it feels like an extraneous activity vis-à-vis the hobby itself. As for the collection it must be reasonably advanced, since it must compete for display space with dealers and other widely recognized leisure collectors.

The same holds for stamp collectors, for which clubs and associations have formed and which have their own regional, national, and international conventions and accompanying exhibitions.[1] Some members of these organizations present a one-off exhibit of an aspect of their collection as an instance of PBL linked to their hobby. In model railroading PBL is also evident as an occasional offshoot of the hobby. It occurs as a display mounted by one or more hobbyists at (usually) a local annual convention or similar gathering of a club of like-minded enthusiasts (Stevens-Ratchford, 2014; Yarwood & Shaw, 2010).

The community in question is family and friends when considering the viewers of collections of home videos and photos. These productions are unique leisure projects to the extent that their content has never been presented in this form by their creators. Furthermore, it is the same kind of community that takes an interest in someone's memoir (Stebbins, 2011). The *Oxford English Dictionary* (fifth ed.) defines a memoir as: "a record of events or history from personal knowledge or from special sources of information; an autobiographical account or (occas.) biographical record." In principle the record referred to here may be written, audio or visual, as in an essay, piece of poetry, recorded oral statement or video-taped account. In practice it is probable that most memoirs are of the essay variety, but with oral and visual types becoming ever more common given advances in and proliferation of facilitative recording equipment. Poetry would seem to be the least popular medium for memoirs, although as shown elsewhere (Stebbins, 2011), seniors can warm to this way of telling about their past. That is, many memoirs are therapeutic audio, visual and written productions created by the elderly, but they can be life histories and autobiographies (all ages) or accounts of personal events (all ages) (Stebbins, 2011). Creating a memoir, as just defined and described, is most commonly a kind of project-based leisure.

Memoirs differ from impromptu, fleeting oral reminiscences, which in most instances are best qualified as casual leisure of the sociable conversation type.

---

[1] Gelber (1992) offers a rich ethnography of stamp collecting as a hobby, albeit without any mention of its hobbyist extensions as PBL.

Memoir-based projects, on the other hand, are free-time activity in which someone works up a record of a major event or, possibly more demanding, of his or her life, an activity that takes time and may require learning certain intellectual and physical skills. The intellectual skills include knowing a language well enough to enable expression of what the person remembers (e.g., sufficient knowledge of vocabulary, sentence construction, paragraph development). The physical skills are evident in an ability to write by hand, use a computer (especially for people unable to write by hand) or operate an audio or video recorder. Nevertheless, these kinds of skill and knowledge would be unnecessary to the extent that someone else does the recording and edits for style and readability what gets registered.

For some serious runners participating in a marathon is PBL. Some of the runners in the study conducted by Ridinger et al. (2012) could well have been engaging in a one-off sampling of their hobby pursued at this intense level. This might be shown to be especially true for the Boston Marathon and other celebrated races of the same distance. Meanwhile, there is another aspect of sports-related volunteering that begets PBL: event volunteering. Thus, Gravelle and Larocque (2005) studied it at an annual edition of the francophone games in Ontario, Canada. Twynam et al. (2002/2003) made similar observations in their study of curling. The event—the Star Choice World Junior Curling Tournament—was held in Thunder Bay, Canada in 1998 and was a one-off occasion for volunteers in that city. The curlers would, for the most part, continue their hobby after the tournament, but not so for the non-curling volunteers. As a third example consider Wilks's (2014) research on volunteers at the 2012 Olympic and Paralympic Games in London and that of Undlien (2019) on people with intellectual disabilities' experiences as volunteers for the Youth Winter Olympic Games held in Lillehammer, Norway in 2016.2.[2]

Sometimes a leisure project becomes truly community-wide, as happened in Exmouth a tiny town (population 3000) in Western Australia hundreds of miles from any city. Tens of thousands descended on it to view the total solar eclipse of April 2023. Natasha Frost (2023) describes how the town successfully organized lodging, portable toilets, food provision, drinking water, entertainment, and more in a singular project centered on the celestial event and the days immediately preceding and following it.

Conclusions

This can happen at an organizational function such as a conference, convention, festival, special exhibition, sports competition, or disaster relief. It can happen when making something, as in constructing housing for Habitat for Volunteering, pure or mixed with amateur or hobbyist interests, is clearly a main way of engaging in

---

[2] Some of the studies mentioned in this paragraph were also cited in Chap. 2 as examples of positive obligatory PBL.

community-related PBL. Humanity in general is the beneficiary of making quilts for a charity (Stalp et al., 2023), while knitting sweaters and mittens for grandchildren, and baking cookies and cakes for the extended family are aimed at much narrower segments of the wider community.

The community involved in genealogical PBL (see Chap. 3) is, mainly, the extended family who will benefit from it and likely contribute to its content and, secondarily, interested outsiders. The genealogist needs information only some of which can be found through impersonal sources such as the Internet and libraries. Thus this enthusiast must also contact by mail, telephone, or face-to-face visits to distant relatives to learn about dates (of birth, death, marriage, etc.), names of offspring, geographic locations, and so on of ancestors.

Public speaking: prepare a talk for a reunion, an after-dinner speech, an oral position statement on an issue to be discussed at a community meeting. In general, the community in question is the audience at these events. And, with the occasional exception of the after-dinner presentation, they are usually one-off leisure involvements, which do nevertheless, require significant preparation and speaking ability.

One last matter remains to be covered in the main part of this book, namely, shared PBL.

References

Carty, M. (2017). What to do when a neighbourhood dog won't stop barking, 8 March 11:53 am, *Globalnews*, https://globalnews.ca/news/3295984.

Case, D. O. (2009). Serial collecting as leisure, and coin collecting in particular. *Library Trends, 57*, 729–752.

Frost, N. (2023). Flocking to one of the few specks of land in sight of a total eclipse. *New York Times* (20 April).

Gelber, S. M. (1992). Free market metaphor: The historical dynamics of stamp collecting. *Comparative Studies in Society and History, 34*(4), 742–769.

Gravelle, F., & Larocque, L. (2005). Volunteerism and serious leisure: The case of the francophone games. *World Leisure Journal, 47*(1), 45–51.

Holmes, K. (2014). 'It fitted in with our lifestyle': An investigation into episodic volunteering in the tourism sector. *Annals of Leisure Research, 17*(4), 443–459.

Macduff, N. L. (1991). *Episodic volunteering: Building the short-term volunteer program.* MBA Publications.

Ridinger, L. L., Funk, D. C., Jordan, J. S., & Kaplanidou, K. (2012). Marathons for the masses: Exploring the role of negotiation-efficacy and involvement on running commitment. *Journal of Leisure Research, 44*(2), 155–178.

Smith, D. H., Stebbins, R. A., & Dover, M. A. (2006). *A dictionary of nonprofit terms and concepts.* Indiana University Press.

Stalp, M. C., Leap, B., & Kelly, K. (2023). 'This was like some *Little House on the Prairie* shit': The intensive care(work) of making PPE during COVID-19. *Journal of Leisure Research.* https://doi.org/10.1080/00222216.2022.2142082

Stebbins, R. A. (2011). Personal memoirs, project-based leisure and therapeutic recreation for seniors, Leisure Reflections, No. 26, *LSA Newsletter*, No. 88, March 2011 (available online at www.seriousleisure.net/Digital Library).

Stevens-Ratchford, R. G. (2014). Serious leisure: A case study of model railroading in relation to successful aging. *Activities, Adaptation and Aging, 38*(2), 113–137.

Twynam, G. D., Farrell, J. M., & Johnston, M. E. (2002/2003). Leisure and volunteer motivation at a special sporting event. *Leisure/Loisir, 27*, 363–377.

Undlien, R. (2019). Lasting social value or a one-off? People with intellectual disabilities' experiences with volunteering for the Youth Olympic Games. *Journal of Sport for Development, 7*(13), 33–45.

Wearing, S. L. (2004). Examining best practice in volunteer tourism. In R. A. Stebbins & M. M. Graham (Eds.), *Volunteering as leisure/leisure as volunteering: An international assessment* (pp. 209–224). CAB International.

Wilks, L. (2014). The lived experience of London 2012 Olympic and Paralympic Games volunteers: A serious leisure perspective. *Leisure Studies, 35*(5), 652–667. https://doi.org/10.1080/02614367.2014.993334

Woodward, S. (2007). Volunteers provide clean water to half a million. *Calgary Herald*, 5 March, p. B2.

Yarwood, R., & Shaw, J. (2010). 'N-gauging' geographies: Craft consumption, indoor leisure and model railways. *Area (Royal Geographical Society), 42*(4), 425–433.

Chapter 5
Sharing Project-Based Leisure

Abstract Many of the PBL activities discussed in this book are undertaken with one or more friends or relatives in the course of which all concerned build or sustain a degree of camaraderie. Still, there are many other projects where this interpersonal sentiment is largely, if not entirely, absent; this is solitary PBL. The latter type is not to be viewed pejoratively, as isolationist activity, but rather seen as an enthusiast's pursuit of a leisure project in the public space. This chapter starts with solitary PBL, which can be done alone in the presence of other people or literally alone without others sharing in it. A project is shared with friends or relatives when they contribute to its realization or benefit from its outcome. Furthermore, project-based leisure is sometimes undertaken for the benefit of others. This is a distinctive form of sharing. In fact, these artefacts are created within the scope of a hobbyist or amateur activity and become PBL by dint of their special link to another person.

Keywords Solitary PBL · Shared PBL · Family · Friends · Recipients of PBL · Audience

Many of the PBL activities discussed in this book are undertaken with one or more friends or relatives in the course of which all concerned build or sustain a degree of camaraderie. Still, there are many other projects where this interpersonal sentiment is largely, if not entirely, absent; this is solitary PBL. The latter type is not to be viewed pejoratively, as isolationist activity, but rather seen as an enthusiast's pursuit of a leisure project in the public space. We start with solitary PBL.

Solitary PBL

One-off leisure projects are sometimes conceived of as a memorable way to get pleasantly involved with one or more friends or relatives who accompany the participant. Examples include a special visit to one's country of origin, dinner at a classy restaurant, visit to a famous museum or historical site, evening of theater or music presented on a celebrated stage, and the like. This type of PBL can also be found in the practical side of life; for instance, the man who constructs a rock garden in his backyard or the woman who volunteers to help with a project having a clear outcome that can be realized in a few weeks (e.g., a bake sale at her children's school).

Some solitary leisure projects, however, can only be done alone. They include a first-time bungee jump, a weekend of meditation and contemplation at a retreat, a solo visit to a special museum exhibit, and the related activities of a student pursuing a degree in a cherished field of study. Certain knot-making hobbies (e.g., knitting (Court, 2019), macramé, quilting (Stalp, 2007), generally interlacing, interlocking, and knot-making from kits) can be a short-term pleasurable activity that can be carried out with little practice and, certainly, can be enjoyed alone (Dirix, 2014; Turney, 2009).

One-off first-time projects are likely to be completed by following ready-made instructions and patterns (available online and described in Pöllänen 2015). The decision to pursue knitting as a hobby, for instance, would therefore seem to come after an initial instructional session, and assuming it is a positive one, there is sufficient free time for it, and costs are reasonable, among other possible constraints. Ordinary reproductive craft involves copying the product from a model. In this case, the maker uses a ready-made design that incorporates the aesthetic or technical qualities, or both, of the artefact. Ordinary craft work can also be a process in which the maker uses a series of technical solutions (using instructions) or reproduces a previously learned model or technique (Pöllänen, 2015, p. 60).

As one-off, single person PBL consider such a project in establishing a club. Thus, Eileen Bostle (1984) describes the emergence of a music and poetry listening club at St. John's hospital, in Stone, near Aylesbury, England, and the County Psychiatric Hospital in Buckinghamshire. The idea behind it sprang from the local library, whose patterns of community use are normal for people outside the hospital, but which must constantly make its presence felt and thereby remain in the forefront of the patients' attention. This is good from the point of view of patients going *out* to the library. The rehabilitation officer at the hospital expressed interest in helping on a regular basis with the listening activities and soon well-known pieces of music of all kinds were being played, interspersed with poems and short stories from spoken word cassettes. The first such session lasted 45 minutes. Club meetings proceeded in a similar fashion for a further 3–4 weeks, at which time a patient asked if he could read out loud from a scrapbook he had been keeping. Toward the end of the same session, one of the patients ask for a specific piece of music to be played the following week, which they had been encouraged to do from the start, though they had left the choice of the piece to the staff. Shortly thereafter the listening club was formally born and would thereafter appear on the hospital occupational therapy timetable. By this time, there were 5 to 6 long-stay patients regularly attending, with the largest number ever to attend being 25 and the lowest 6. At this point, according to Bostle, the activity took on its final form. At the end of each session the patients in the group would discuss which items of music they would like the following week and, if they were not available in the library's cassette collection, attempts would be made through the following week to obtain them from the local record library or to borrow them from someone in the local community.

Sean O'Riada's desire to form an Irish folk music group illustrates further this variety of PBL. He discussed his plan with Hazel Fairbairn (1994), posing the question of what kind of musicians he should have. Fairbairn suggested he should very definitely have Sonnie Brogan and John Kelly, since they were old traditional musicians and would certainly know all the old tunes. Moreover, they would soon tell him if he was doing something radically wrong according to traditional music standards. In forming this group O'Riada tried to incorporate into the arrangements the learning processes and performance skills of respected traditional players, an inspiration born of his own background in western art music composition. His idea was to incorporate the variation of the monodic line, which he perceived as central to traditional music-making, into a structure which maximized the textural variety offered by the group context. His first aim was to counteract the "musical abomination" of the ceili band sound (a type of Irish folk music). But his ideas met with significant resistance from the traditional players. As argued by analysts in this field, the ceili band has its roots in the fundamental aspect of the instrumental tradition, in that the music is tailored to the needs of dancers. As far as the dancer is concerned, lift and good rhythm are more important than variation. Contrary to O Riada's view, some individual ornamentation and nuances of melodic interpretation can be heard in regional-based bands like The Tulla and The Kilfenora. These bands have also produced many fine traditional solo players. Nevertheless, O'Riada finally won the support of the musicians with whom he worked, owing to his willingness to integrate his compositional creativity (on the level of the arrangement) with the restraints of traditional style (on the level of melodic variation and ornamentation).

Ben MacIntyre (2022) explores in his recent book some incredible PBL at Colditz, the Nazi's Fortress Prison of World War II, which was established in an old German castle. One inventive project features a tiny Scotsman who, hidden in an old mattress, sneaks up to the glider he built entirely inside the castle attic as part of his plan to fly in it from the roof. MacIntyre notes that once on the ground the escapee made it by foot in May 1941 to the then-neutral American consulate in Vienna. Here an official refused to help in any way, saying: "They'll get you in the end. They always do."

Shared PBL

A project is shared with friends or relatives when they contribute to its realization or benefit from its outcome. These co-participants are evident in myriad projects examined below under the headings of family and friends. We turn first to those in the participant's family.

Family Co-Participants

A prominent type is the many mother-daughter, father-son projects including those where the parent is instead a grandparent. Possibly the best known PBL here is mother and daughter collaborating to bake a cake or batch of cookies (assuming that sharing this activity is infrequent for the two participants). Father and son (now at least in his mid-teens) might together go on a special fishing or hunting trip.

And whole families sometimes arrange their own PBL, it often being of the tourist kind. For instance, a family might spend a couple of weeks in the country from which the parents recently emigrated. Festivals are often attended as PBL, as one-off samplings of music (e.g., folk, jazz), theater [e.g., the fringe festivals (see http://www.worldfringe.com/members), Shakespearian works (see https://nosweatshakespeare.com/festivals), or comedy festivals (see https://thecomicscomic.com/comedy-festivals)]. These are family entertainment, but generally only so for adult members. Before moving on to the next section, remember the case presented in Chap. 2 as opportune PBL. It was the 107-day canoe trip made by a family of four (including two children) through the western Northwest Territories of Canada, which also serves as a vivid example of shared PBL (Strong, 2022).

Sharaievska and Mirehie (2023) explore the use of social media before, during and after family trips, to send communications that tend to feature the positive sites and experiences seen and felt by touring friends and relatives. The content of these messages are typically cell-phone photos of people and places (selfies included) and running annotative commentary as the trip progresses. Afterward, some members of this "audience" may be invited to a slide show of the trip's highlights presented on a much larger screen than that of a cell phone.

A Birthday Slide Show[1]

Peggy's sixtieth birthday was 3 months off, when three members of her immediate family decided to stage a surprise party to celebrate the occasion in grand fashion. A division of labor was struck, in which father would book a restaurant and invite the guests, while the son and one of the daughters would assemble a detailed slide show of Peggy's life, running from her birth to the present. With 25 guests and the need to invite them secretly, father was undertaking some project-based leisure of his own (best classified as informal volunteering). Nonetheless, the project of his two children was even more complicated and time-consuming, and for these reasons, is the one on which we will concentrate here.

To build their slide show (entertainment theatre project), they had to contact maternal relatives in distant parts of the country to obtain copies of earlier photographs of Peggy and of important people and events in her life. This material was

---

[1] This section taken from Stebbins (2005, p. 7).

then assembled into a chronological account of her main work and leisure activities up to her sixtieth year. Some specialized background knowledge was required to create the slide show, for it was to be projected by computer. So, it fell to Peggy's son to attend to this facet of the project, while her daughter saw to rounding up the photographs and developing a story line.

The show consisted of 180 slides, which were presented in a 45-min session following the dinner. Peggy, from whom the entire event had been successfully kept secret, was flabbergasted by it all.

Friends as Co-Participants

Several of the kinds of family co-participation in PBL can also be undertaken with friends, namely, baking, hunting and fishing trips, attending festivals, and trips into the wilderness. All of these can be one-off leisure projects, and they include back-packing adventures (with an experienced leader), easy leader-guided mountain ascents (e.g., Kilimanjaro, beginners' routes with guide; Mt. Fuji, easiest route with some prior conditioning), and canoe/kayak trips (see online websites). Most common, however, are the one-off tourism projects to famous cities and regions. Most of these are commercially guided train, bus, and river or canal tours (defined as casual leisure, Stebbins, 1996). Cultural tourism to these cities and regions, which when pursued as a hobby, is serious leisure, and is more likely than its casual counterpart to be self-organized. Both types can be experienced with family or with friends.

Some ocean cruises and road trips whether with family or friends (or both) offer another kind of shared PBL. The Internet contains a wide sampling of these two types. Additionally, *Lonely Planet* publishes a number of guides describing road trips in various parts the world. Each such trip is a project in itself, but is not PBL if this kind of touring is an enduring hobby. For example, a retired couple in Canada has plans to spend 2 weeks in the spring in Scandinavia, a week in late summer in the Seattle area, and visit New Zealand in November. This is enduring tourism, with PBL being experienced in each mini-project pursued during each tour (e.g., in Scandinavia visiting Stockholm, Oslo, Bergen, and Copenhagen). One such mini-project might be to visit a well-known museum in the destination city (e.g., Cerdan Chiscano, 2023).

Punch and Snellgrove (2023) point out nevertheless that such projects can be scenes of dissention as well of those of concord. They found that touring couples were sometimes unequally attracted to certain events or sites for myriad reasons, among them physical setting (too crowded, poor sightlines, bad acoustics), offensive content (too dirty, insulting), unattractive content (boring, too riské, low quality material), and the like. The two authors studied the ways in which their subjects negotiate their differences along these lines and other disagreements.

Recipients of PBL

Project-based leisure is sometimes undertaken for the benefit of others. This is a distinctive form of sharing. Thus, knitting a sweater for somebody is shared PBL, as is making a chair or painting a landscape for a relative or friend. In fact, these artefacts are created within the scope of a hobbyist or amateur activity and become PBL by dint of their special link to another person. Outside such personal giving the products of these enthusiasts are sold in the broader, impersonal marketplace, like Etsy (online marketing of visual arts and crafts), community craft fairs, and local galleries. Or they may be donated to a charity, to family or friends as gifts (not requested), offered at auctions or on consignment (e.g., https://www.artsy.net/sell), and the like.

Still, many products are never sold, donated, or given away, but instead are stored by their creators in their residence, studio, atelier, and so on. Upon their death or incapacity due to old age, the fate of these creations now lies in the hands of that person's heirs. The community landfill may be the ultimate destination of some of these items.

Pamela Reynolds (2018) describes the artist's problem in greater detail.

> There's a dirty little secret among artists. It can be summed up this way: We create art. Our art does not sell. We stuff the art in our closets.
>
> Before long, our closets are filled, so we turn to storage bins. Those fill up quickly too, so we resort to corners of our studios. If our studios aren't large enough, we cart our paintings and our *objets d'art* to our homes where they quickly occupy every surface, both horizontal and vertical. Pretty soon, we are buried.
>
> We learn inventive ways to handle art overload. We begin working smaller. We switch from canvas to paper. We move from sculpture to painting, from painting to drawing, from drawing to photography.
>
> Others, like me, reach a crisis point. I am a fairly prolific painter with boxes of paintings wedged tight just about anywhere you might look, but I must decide what to do with my art before the camera crew of "Hoarders" comes knocking at my studio door.
>
> Should I recycle all my older work by painting over old canvases? Destroy all my old canvases altogether? Give them away? *(And hey, wait a moment, how can I sell paintings and give them away at the same time?)* Then, I wrestle with even greater existential questions. Should I even be producing new work at all, given the state of our planet? Somehow, it seems irresponsible to be adding more things, no matter how beautiful, to a world in which giant garbage patches drift aimlessly around our oceans. I pride myself on many things when it comes to my carbon footprint. I don't eat meat. I don't own a car. But here I am with my carbon shoe size growing larger every time I order more art supplies from Dick Blick.
>
> I don't eat meat. I don't own a car. But here I am with my carbon shoe size growing larger every time I order more art supplies from Dick Blick.
>
> Boston-based artist John Vinton has confronted this problem and found a solution. First, it must be said, Vinton is one of the lucky ones. He paints about 15–20 canvases a year and sells, he estimates, about 80% of them. But, as all artists know, there is one big caveat.
>
> "It's very inconsistent," he admits. "And it does create a problem with some pieces. My preferred solution is to make room by taking canvases off stretchers and rolling them. But on some of my pieces where the paint is really built up, I'm a little concerned about doing that, because the paint could crack."

That means, like the rest of us, Vinton gets stuck with artistic build-up. Although he loves to work large on imposing canvases that might span 5 or 6 feet across (and he would work even larger if he had the space for it), he has allowed his artistic expression to cede to cold, hard practicalities.

"I do like working large, but I've sort of gotten myself more into working at a smaller scale because they're easier to store," says Vinton. "You can do a whole bunch of small ones, and if they don't sell, it's not that big of a deal." This month, he moved into a smaller studio in the same building, so the problem is likely to become more acute.

Conclusions

I noted at the beginning of this chapter that many of the PBL activities discussed in this book are undertaken with one or more friends or relatives in the course of which all concerned build or sustain a degree of camaraderie. This is a main source of the well-being experienced while engaged in PBL. Successfully completing a project is another such source and perhaps the only one for solitary projects. Of course, the greater the complexity of a project and the amount of time needed to complete it the greater the feeling of well-being resulting therefrom.

One way to continue along this road to personal development is to explore turning a PBL activity into a serious pursuit.

References

Bostle, E. (1984). The listening club: A poetry and music activity. *Health Librairies Review, 1*, 209–212.

Cerdan Chiscano, M. (2023). Co-creating family-inclusive leisure experiences: A study of Barcelona's Gran Teatre del Liceu opera house. *Journal of Leisure Research*. https://doi.org/10.1080/00222216.2023.2187265

Court, K. (2019). Knitting two together (k2tog), "if you meet another knitter you always have a friend". *Textile: The Journal of Cloth and Culture, 18*(3), 278–291. https://doi.org/10.1080/14759756.2019.1690838

Dirix, E. (2014). Stitched up – Representations of contemporary vintage style mania and the darkside of the popular knitting revival. *Textile: Journal of Cloth and Culture, 12*(1), 86–99.

MacIntyre, B. (2022). *Prisoners of the castle: An epic story of survival and escape from Colditz, the Nazis' Fortress Prison*. Penguin Random House Canada.

Pöllänen, S. (2015). Craft as leisure-based coping strategy: Craft makers' descriptions of their stress-reducing activity. *Occupational Therapy in Mental Health, 31*(2), 83–100. https://doi.org/10.1080/0164212X.2015.1024377

Punch, S., & Snellgrove, M. (2023). Bridging time: Negotiating serious leisure in intimate couple relationships. *Annals of Leisure Research*. https://doi.org/10.1080/11745398.2023.2197243

Reynolds, P. (2018). *With all the canvases*. Accessed March 23, 2023, from https://www.wbur.org/news/2018/03/27/artist-dilemma-art-overload (27 March).

Sharaievska, I., & Mirehie, M. (2023). Use of social media before, during and after family trips. *Journal of Leisure Research*. https://doi.org/10.1080/00222216.2023.2182165

Stalp, M. B. (2007). *Quilting: The fabric of everyday life*. Berg.

Stebbins, R. A. (1996). Cultural tourism as serious leisure. *Annals of Tourism Research, 23*, 948–950.

Stebbins, R. A. (2005). Project-based leisure: Theoretical neglect of a common use of free time. *Leisure Studies, 24*, 1–11.

Strong, W. (2022). Family of 4 makes 1500 km journey through N.W.T. backcountry. *CBC News* (22 September). Accessed October 15, 2022, from https://www.cbc.ca/news/canada/north/nwt-backcountry-travel-with-youngsters-1.5292099

Turney, J. (2009). *The culture of knitting*. Berg.

Chapter 6
Conclusion

Abstract The most obvious conclusion to emerge from this book is the need for more research on the immense variety of PBL in our time. There is also some conceptual work that remains to be done, notably, to separate more sharply the somewhat skilled/knowledgeable PBL from hobbies pursued along the same lines. This can be accomplished by way of qualitative research on particular activities that are taken up either as projects or as hobbyist or amateur activities. First, however, we must sharpen the distinction between non-work obligation and project-based leisure. Obligation and leisure would, at first glance, seem to be exact opposites. Yet, if the word "volunteering" is to remain consistent with its French and Latin roots, then it can only be seen, as all leisure is, as un-coerced, activity. Moreover, as with all leisure, leisure volunteering can only be seen as either a basically satisfying or as a basically deeply rewarding experience.

Keywords Qualitative research · Obligation · Volunteering · Interstitial leisure · Level of skill and knowledge · Dabbling · Eudaimonism

The most obvious conclusion to emerge from this book is the need for more research on the immense variety of PBL in our time. There is also some conceptual work that remains to be done, notably, to separate more sharply the somewhat skilled/knowledgeable PBL from hobbies pursued along the same lines. This can be accomplished by way of qualitative research on particular activities that are taken up either as projects or as hobbyist or amateur activities.

First, however, we must sharpen the distinction between non-work obligation and project-based leisure.

The Role of Obligation in Leisure

Obligation and leisure would, at first glance, seem to be exact opposites. Leisure is experienced in free time, whereas obligatory activity is coerced, not free. Consider volunteering as a case in point (see Chap. 4). Failure to recognize that some people volunteer out of a sense of responsibility, out of a sense of obligation that is, nonetheless, negatively felt. In other words, such volunteers would rather pass their free time in bona fide leisure activities, which are positive in nature. Negatively obligated volunteering has been conceptualized as a kind of non-work obligation (Stebbins 2015, p. 7, 2000, 2021a).

If the word "volunteering" is to remain consistent with its French and Latin roots, then it can only be seen, as all leisure is, as un-coerced, activity. Moreover, as with all leisure, leisure volunteering can only be seen as either a basically satisfying or as a basically deeply rewarding experience. Otherwise, we are forced to posit that so-called volunteers of this kind are somehow pushed into performing their roles by circumstances they would prefer to avoid—a stark contradiction of terms.

By the way, this clarification should help sort out what true volunteering is in non-European societies (Polus et al., 2023). In other words, how much of non-work activity there is not coerced by custom, by negative obligations, and the like. Note, too, that volunteering is conceptualized in volunteer studies as conducted only beyond the interests of the volunteer's immediate family; obligation versus non-obligation being too difficult to separate conceptually at this intimate level.

Furthermore, I wrote nearly 25 years ago (Stebbins, 2000) that positive, or agreeable, obligation is possible in all three domains of the SLP. Obligation is not about people being prevented from entering certain leisure activities—see the research on leisure constraints—but about people failing to define a given activity as leisure or redefining it as other than leisure, that is, as an unpleasant obligation, if not both of these. Moreover, obligation is both a micro-level state of mind, an attitude—a person feels obligated—and a form of behavior—he must carry out a particular course of action, engage in a particular activity. But even while obligation is substantially mental and behavioral, it roots, too, in the social and cultural world of the obligated actor. Consequently, we may even speak of a macro-level of culture of obligation that takes shape around many a work, leisure, and non-work activity (Stebbins, 2017, p. 30).

Obligation relates to leisure in at least two ways: leisure may include certain agreeable obligations and the third domain of life—non-work obligation—consists of disagreeable requirements capable of limiting the positiveness that can be experienced in free time. Agreeable obligation is a main feature of some leisure, especially evident when this kind of obligation accompanies positive commitment to an activity capable of arousing pleasant memories and expectations (these two are essential features of leisure, Kaplan, 1960, pp. 22–25). Nevertheless, it could also be argued that agreeable obligation in leisure is never really felt as such, because the participant is eager to pursue the activity in any case.

Finally, PBL enhances one's optimal leisure lifestyle and thereby one's sense of well-being. This adds the icing to the cake of well-being.

Moreover, it appears that in some instances project-based leisure spring from a sense of obligation to undertake it. If so it is nonetheless done as leisure, as un-coerced activity, in the sense that the obligation is in fact "agreeable"—the project creator in executing the project anticipates finding fulfillment, obligated or not. And worth exploring, given that some obligations can be pleasant and attractive, is the nature and extent of leisure-like projects carried out as part of paid employment. Furthermore, this discussion jibes with the additional criterion that the project, to qualify as project-based leisure, must be *seen by the project creator* as fundamentally un-coerced, fulfilling activity. Finally, note that project-based leisure cannot, by definition, refer to projects executed as part of a person's serious leisure. Examples include mounting a star night as an amateur astronomer or a model train display as a hobbyist.

Though not serious leisure, project-based leisure is enough like it to justify using the serious leisure perspective to develop a parallel framework for exploring this class of activities. A primary difference is that project-based leisure fails to imbue participants with a sense of career. Otherwise, however, there is need here to persevere, acquire in some cases certain skills or knowledge and, invariably, put out some effort. Also present are recognizable benefits, a special identity, and often a social world of sorts. Although the latter it appears is usually less complicated than those in which most serious leisure activities are framed. And it may happen at times that, even when not intended at the moment as participation in a type of serious leisure, the skilled, artistic, or intellectual aspects of the project prove highly attractive. Realizing this, the participant decides after the fact to make a leisure career of the activity as a hobbyist, amateur, or career volunteer pursuit (see Stebbins 2014, see Chap. 2 and Fig. 2.1).

Project-based leisure is also capable of generating many of the rewards experienced in serious leisure. And, as in serious leisure so in project-based leisure: these rewards constitute part of the motivational basis for engaging in such highly fulfilling activity. Furthermore, motivation to undertake a leisure project may have an organizational base, much as many other forms of leisure do. My observations suggest that small groups, grassroots associations (volunteer groups with few or no paid staff), and volunteer organizations (paid-staff groups using volunteer help) are the most common types of organizations in which people undertake project-based leisure.

Motivationally speaking, project-based leisure may be attractive in substantial part because it, unlike serious leisure, rarely demands long-term commitment. Even occasional projects carry with them the sense that the undertaking in question has a definite end. Indeed, it may even be terminated prematurely. Thus project-based leisure is not what Robert Dubin (1992) called a "central life interest." Rather it is viewed by participants as fulfilling (as distinguished from enjoyable or hedonic) activity that can be experienced comparatively quickly, though certainly not as quickly as most casual leisure.

Project-based leisure fits into leisure lifestyle in its own peculiar way as interstitial activity. In this it resembles some casual leisure but not most serious leisure. Project-based leisure can therefore help shape a person's optimal leisure lifestyle. For instance, it can often be pursued at times convenient for the participant. It follows that project-based leisure is nicely suited to people who, out of proclivity or extensive non-leisure obligations or both, reject serious leisure and, yet, who also have no appetite for a steady diet of casual leisure. Among the candidates for project-based leisure are people with heavy workloads; homemakers, mothers, and fathers with extensive domestic responsibilities; unemployed individuals who, though looking for work, still have time at the moment for (I suspect, mostly one-shot) projects; and avid serious leisure enthusiasts who want a temporary change in their leisure lifestyle. Retired people who often do have time for discretionary activity may find project-based leisure attractive as a way of adding spice and variety to their lifestyles. Beyond these special categories of participant, project-based leisure offers a form of substantial leisure to all adults, adolescents, and even children looking for something interesting and exciting to do in free time that is neither casual nor serious leisure.

And, lest it be overlooked, note that one-off projects also hold the possibility of becoming unpleasant. Thus, the hobbyist genealogist gets overwhelmed with the details of family history and the challenge of verifying dates. The thought of putting in time and effort doing something once considered leisure but which she now dislikes makes no sense. Likewise, volunteering for a project may turn sour. The volunteer is now faced with a disagreeable obligation, which however, must still be honored. This is leisure no more.

Level of Skill and Knowledge

Acquiring a level of skill and knowledge sufficient to finish decently a leisure project as opposed to that needed for routine hobbyist or amateur activity amount to two different personal developments. For one, the project is unlikely to require the breadth of skill and knowledge that a leisure career in an art or craft does. Thus, learning and presenting a part in a play as a one-off project fails to equip the serious amateur with many of the theatrical skills and wide experiential background needed to perform in a variety of dramatic works. The same can be said for painting. For it is one thing to complete a landscape in an introductory art class and quite another to become able to paint decently a wide variety of landscapes (as a continuous set of amateur projects).

A similar hobbyist career might unfold for those who construct furniture from a kit [e.g., Chad Stanton's (2018) book]. Having developed a taste for working with wood by way of a project kit, this newly minted enthusiast decides to build a desk with drawers now guided only by a set of plans. Some new tools may need to be purchased or borrowed, but this person is now familiar with these kinds of implements rather than being wary of them. Finally, consider the fan who buys a poster commemorating an annual jazz festival, constituting thus a simple consumer project. Enamored of this purchase this person strives to become a collector of past and future posters advertising this festival. Such hobbyists commonly develop a rich knowledge about the artists of these works, the music and musicians referred to in them, the history of the festival in question, and so on (On the hobby and PBL of poster collecting, see https://www.google.com/search?client=firefox-b-d&q=poster+collecting; https://www.allposters.com.)

Fulfillment careers are born in particular activities enjoyed in daily life, where from time to time, people explore the vast world of free-time interests. Typically, these beginnings are prosaic, especially compared with the participant's career when fulfilment is at its apogee. This is not to say that such careers inevitably reach the heights of those enjoyed by the best movie stars, sports heroes, successful small-business people, or respected trades workers. Nevertheless, no one seeking a fulfilment career *starts* out at the top.

The purpose of this section is to examine the key processes and conditions that facilitate embarking on a fulfillment career. One of them is accidental discovery, discussed here as dabbling. Another is memorable contact with an exemplar of the work/leisure activity on which such a career is founded. Both processes may inspire some strategic planning, arranging for deeper learning, and parallel participation as a neophyte.

PBL as Dabbling

So far as the study of leisure is concerned, 'dabbler' first appeared as a scientific concept in 1979 (Stebbins, 1979, pp. 20, 30). Then, as now, dabbling has been conceived of as a kind of play, which starting with my conceptualization, was classified as one type of casual leisure (Stebbins, 1982, 1997). The amateur-professional-public system of relationships, introduced in my 1979 book, placed the dabbler as part of the public of the other two, as someone who is from time to time amused while trying to emulate performance of a given art, sport, or entertainment activity. But a real performance it is not, for by definition the dabbler lacks the training and practice needed for this.

This view of the dabbler—as part of a public—has tended to obscure this leisure participant's broader relationship with the amateurs and professionals. Fortunately, development of the SLP has given us in a more encompassing theoretic orientation. It encourages and facilitates seeing in as rich detail as possible the many ways in which dabblers, amateurs, hobbyists, professionals, and most recently, project-based leisure enthusiasts are related.

The proposition that dabbling is the first step taken by some great professionals in launching their careers may seem preposterous. It can be hard to imagine an accomplished pianist having once hesitantly tapped out notes on a keyboard or a famous soccer player having once clumsily kicked a ball around a local park. By no means all professional careers originate in this kind of play but, for those that do disinterestedness is, ironically, the attitude that precedes deep commitment to the serious pursuit.

As just noted dabbling is a kind of play. More particularly, it is spontaneous activity engaged in for its own sake, for curiosity and hedonic experience. It is 'disinterested' in the sense that no long-term goal is envisioned while dabbling; the participant simply wants certain immediate experiences (this conceptualization of play is that of Johan Huizinga (1955). Furthermore, these experiences need not be physical, as they usually are for example in music and certain outdoor activities, but can be mental such as in flights of imagination triggered through reading (Stebbins, 2013).

Dabbling and the CL-SL Continuum

Nonetheless, some people do dabble at an activity, and a proportion of this group moves on to pursuing it more seriously as a neophyte. Yet, dabbling is impossible in certain activities, forcing would-be enthusiasts to start as neophytes. Here, to learn of their affinity for it, they must actually undertake some careful preparation. Whether people embark on their fulfillment careers indirectly as dabblers or directly as neophytes, they do so within a serious pursuit. Scientific discussion of this transition has come to be known as the "CL-SL [casual-serious leisure] Continuum." A central question here has revolved around whether casual leisure dabbling is a precursor to becoming a neophyte in a serious pursuit. The preceding observations suggest that this happens adventitiously, only in certain kinds of activities, and only for participants who want to get serious about their leisure.

Thus fulfilment careers begin with becoming a neophyte in that pursuit (Stebbins, 2014, p. 31). Being a neophyte means, among other things, signalling to self, and often, certain other people the intention to get better at it. This is achieved along the lines of four fundamental dimensions: effort, skill, knowledge, and experience. Gains along these four, as they apply to the activity in question, put the participant on the road to personal development, self-fulfillment, and a career in the activity. Neophytes manifest their intention to get better by engaging in such formative activities as taking lessons, reading extensively, practicing fundamental skills, observing experienced participants, and the like.

Neophytes are not casual leisure participants. Even the erstwhile dabblers have moved away from their hedonic interest in the activity. Still, the fact that some neophytes have been attracted earlier to the activity purely for its raw enjoyment is not to be ignored. Examples include the child who taps out chop sticks and other ditties on the piano and later becomes interested in piano lessons; the back garden star gazer using a cheap telescope who decides to get more serious by joining the local astronomy club; the joke-telling life of the party who, wanting to become a stand-up comic, mounts an "open-mic" stage, and with that launches a career in the art. The fulfillment career begins with a neophyte level of interest in the activity, but the casual dabbling as these examples show can be a crucial precursor. If priming the pump is what makes the pump work, then the priming cannot be dismissed as a minor step in the process.

Conclusions

Finding an interesting project to do in the interstices of free time can be a challenge, especially if some of the former can last as long as a month or more. The latter are not commonly so long. Nevertheless, bridging the diverse gaps in which leisure projects can spark noticeable enthusiasm is worth the effort. In other words, they, too, contribute to subjective well-being. Karl Wallenda, the great high-wire performer, observed that "life is on the wire, the rest is just waiting" (Wikipedia, Karl Wallenda, retrieved 8 July 2023). For Wallenda "the rest" presumably consisted of his leisure interstices, periods of his existence not devoted to high-wire performance and preparing for it or to nonwork obligations (Stebbins, 2021b).

Hamilton-Smith (1995, pp. 6–7) held that our lack of knowledge about the link between serious leisure and well-being is a major lacuna in contemporary leisure research. Recently I observed (Stebbins, 2021c) that 25 years later we are finally starting to tackle this gap, as carried out in Lee and Hwang's (2018) confirmatory study of serious leisure and social well-being and that of Sheldon, Corcoran, and Prentice (2018) who compare hedonic and eudaimonic well-being. They found that education, personal enrichment, individual self-expression, and self-gratification and enjoyment were significant predictors of social well-being. In general, demographic factors accounted for a small percentage of the variance in social well-being, whereas the serious leisure's six qualities showed noticeably more explanatory power.

Project-based leisure also has its eudaimonic properties, even if fewer of them and with less intensity for each. It thereby contributes to well-being—i.e., it helps optimize our experience of it—leaving to those whose leisure lifestyle is anchored in one or more serious leisure activities the enviable feeling of having found an optimal leisure lifestyle.

References

Dubin, R. (1992). *Central life interests: Creative individualism in a complex world*. Transaction.

Hamilton-Smith, E. (1995, March 4–9). The connexions of scholarship. *Newsletter* (Official newsletter of RC13 of the International Sociological Association.

Huizinga, J. (1955). *Homo ludens: A study of the play element in culture*. Beacon.

Kaplan, M. (1960). *Leisure in America: A social inquiry*. Wiley.

Lee, K. J., & Hwang, S. (2018). Serious leisure qualities and subjective well-being. *Journal of Positive Psychology, 13*(1), 48–56. https://doi.org/10.1080/17439760.2017.1374437

Polus, R., Carr, N., & Walters, T. (2023). Challenging the Eurocentrism in volunteering. *World Leisure Journal, 65*(1), 101–118. https://doi.org/10.1080/16078055.2022.2146741

Sheldon, K., Corcoran, M., & Prentice, M. (2018). Pursuing eudaimonic functioning versus pursuing hedonic well-being: The first goal succeeds in its aim, whereas the second does not. *Journal of Happiness Studies*. https://doi.org/10.1007/s10902-018-9980-4

Stanton, C. (2018). *I can do that -- Furniture projects*. Penguin.

Stebbins, R. A. (1979). *Amateurs: On the margin between work and leisure*. Sage. (also available at www.seriousleisure.net/Digital Library)

Stebbins, R. A. (1982). Serious leisure: A conceptual statement. *Pacific Sociological Review, 25*, 251–272.

Stebbins, R. A. (1997). Casual leisure: A conceptual statement. *Leisure Studies, 16*, 17–25.

Stebbins, R. A. (2000). Obligation as an aspect of leisure experience. *Journal of Leisure Research, 32*, 152–155.

Stebbins, R. A. (2013). *The committed reader: Reading for utility, pleasure, and fulfillment in the twenty-first century*. Scarecrow Press.

Stebbins, R. A. (2014). *Careers in serious leisure: From dabbler to devotee in search of fulfillment*. Palgrave Macmillan.

Stebbins, R. A. (2015). *Leisure and the motive to volunteer: Theories of serious, casual, and project-based leisure*. Palgrave Macmillan.

Stebbins, R. A. (2017). *Leisure activities in context: A micro-macro/agency-structure interpretation of leisure*. Transaction/New York, Routledge.

Stebbins, R. A. (2021a). Volunteering and obligation: Positive and negative. In K. Holmes, L. Lockstone-Binney, K. A. Smith, & R. Shipway (Eds.), *Routledge handbook of volunteering in events, sport and tourism* (pp. 425–433). Routledge.

Stebbins, R. A. (2021b). *Non-work obligations: On the delicate art of dealing with disagreeableness*. Emerald Group.

Stebbins, R. A. (2021c). When leisure engenders health: Fragile effects and precautions. *Annals of Leisure Research, 24*(3), 430–444.